The Stepping Stones to Healthy Body and Mind

The Benefits of Ayurveda and Intermittent Fasting

Book One:

The Healing of Ayurveda
Ayurvedic Remedies for the Three Dosha Types

Book Two:

The Definitive Guide of Intermittent Fasting

How to Benefit from Fasting and is it for Everyone

The Healing of Ayurveda

Ayurvedic Remedies for the Three Dosha Types

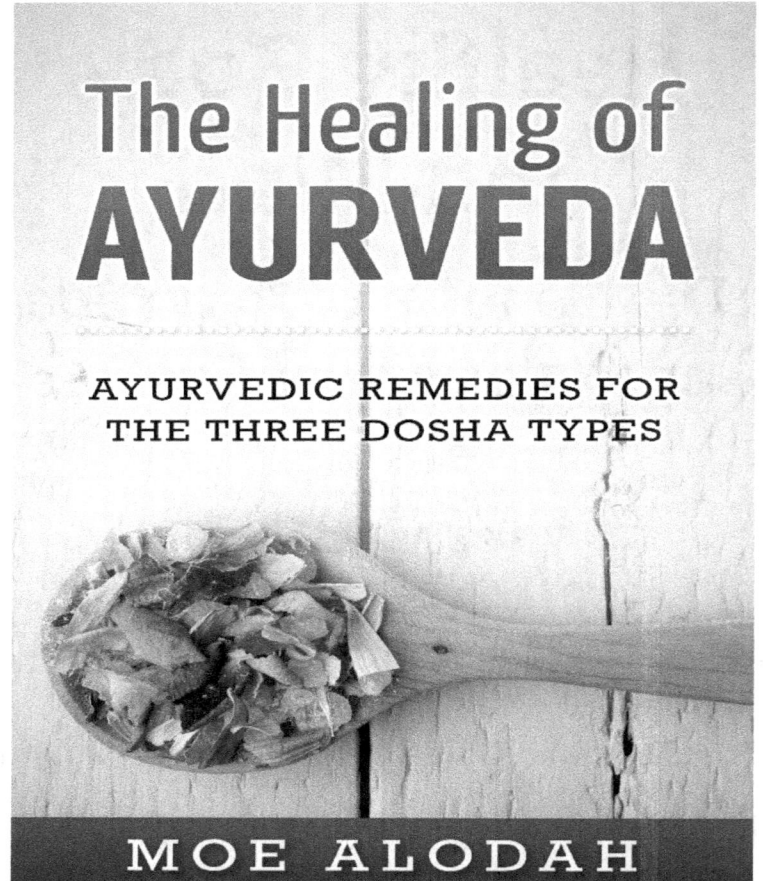

Table of content

INTRODUCTION

Ayurvedic Remedies of the Three Dosha Type

The health of an individual depends on the coordination of both the living and non-living components of the universe. The state of balance between the body, spirit, and mind will determine whether one is of good health or not. Due to this, Indians discovered Ayurveda, a medical strategy that was aimed at harmonizing the mind, spirit, and body for quality functioning. In western nations like the United States, this approach helps as a supplement medication or as a substitute for the common medical practices.

Ayurveda is a holistic healing technique that creates coordination of all the elements of life. The principles that guide the ayurvedic therapy aim at promoting health rather than treatment of the conditions. The therapy is an all-encompassing approach. Factors like the genetic defects, injuries, emotions and age will all affect the balance of life components within the universe. The elements in the universe combine to form three doshas. The Vata, Pitta, and Kapha doshas are inherent with only a single mix dominant in an individual. The balance of the life energies is responsible for sickness or health of a person.

For Ayurveda, the doshas test is vital in determining the outstanding element combinations in a person. Prevention of a condition depends on the dosha combination of an individual. How we sleep, eat and all the other health practices will depend on the dominant combination of the five life elements. It is, therefore, important we assess our life energies balance before any ayurvedic action. Qualified practitioners are the only ones capable of accurately analyzing the doshas from different people. Simple self-tests are available online to help in the determination of your correct element combinations for a healthy living.

The use of herbs in health promotion is not a directive as per the ethics of Ayurveda. They, however, help in maintaining the desired balance of the life elements to avoid the resultant health defects. Different plants have proven to be of benefit in maintaining a correct state of dynamic in the promotion of natural healing. In addition to the herbs, some recipes maintain the balance of the specific dosha. Health is, therefore, a balance between the state of mind, body and spirit.

CHAPTER ONE: What Is Ayurveda

Natural healing is what every person would desire in the case of body dysfunction. This will only be possible when states of the body, mind, and spirit are constant. This means that health is not just the absence of disease or infirmity but includes the dynamic states of all the responsible elements.

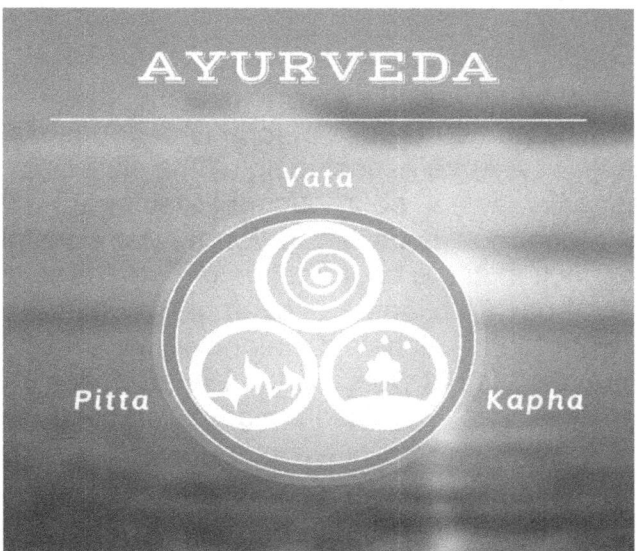

Thousands of years back, Indians applied Ayurveda, an intervention thought to induce the natural healing process of the body. According to this philosophy, the five key elements in the universe (space, fire, earth, water and air) manifest within a person in a unique manner. Every individual has his or her own outstanding combinations. The components responsible combine in threes to form a distinctive dosha combination in different individuals.

Why Ayurveda is considered an individualized health benefit

People have varying dosha combinations. This means that for a productive ayurvedic remedies, each person has to identify his or her specific combination. This also helps in determining the likelihood of a subject contracting certain health conditions. Any individual aiming to live a healthy life should consider some important factors:

1. Proper eating habit
Ingesting food with medical awareness is the key to a healthy life. The prime purpose of food is to nourish our bodies. With Ayurveda, including all the six basic food tastes (salty, sweet, sour, pungent, astringent and bitter) in one meal is preferred. Each taste has its own prime function in the coordination of both the mind and the body functions. For example, regulated intake of sweet foods will help in balancing the Vata and the Pitta doshas but worsens the Kapha dosha when taken in excess. This also brings satisfaction to the body.

Including all the tastes in our diet will help us take all the useful nutrients into our bodies. The feeling of satisfaction will dominate your body without the urge to engage in snacking, which is one of the contributing factors for lifestyle conditions like obesity.

2. Adequate rest
One principle of the Ayurveda is the interconnection between the mind and the body. Adequate sleeping time will make your mind relax as well as boosting the immune functioning. A minimum of six hours sleeping time will make you wake up active and strong for the

day's task. Self-relaxing practices like taking a light meal before going to bed are recommendable for a restful night.

3. Knowledge about your specific dosha
Denoted by the Ayurveda, a personalized approach to health, knowing the combination of elements responsible for your unique dosha is important in knowing the individualized actions to enhance your wellbeing. Knowing your class will help you know the specific needs to stay healthy.
In any intervention or project, there must be some guiding principles. The Ayurveda has some principles that when taken into consideration, will lead to a longer life:

- The philosophy views health in the three doshas. Like mentioned above, knowing your life energies will be of great help when undertaking the health intervention programs. The three doshas are detailed in the next chapter.

- The actions of the Ayurveda are based on the preventive healthcare principle. However, in western nations, this program supplements the existing healthcare practices.

- The medication aims at providing the first-line protection against infections. The traditional use of neti pot against respiratory infections is a good illustration of prevention at the source. This prevents inhaling pollutants into the respiratory system. It is considered a natural breathing support.

- Boosting the digestive system is one way the ancient Ayurveda works. Good health depends on the capability of our body to metabolize nutrients and eliminate the wastes from the system. Practices like introducing the six tastes in our diet will support the digestive fire.

- The fact that every individual has a unique life energy means that the acquisition of state of balance within the body will vary from person to person. The spirit, body, and mind coordinate to define our health. The distinctive combination of the elements in a person will also describe their wellbeing.

CHAPTER TWO: What Are The Three Dosha Types?

Fire, space, earth, air and water are the matters that characterize the universe. Our health depends on how our body interact with these substances. The elements are described depending on how we experience them. Like said earlier, health of an individual depends on the holistic roles of both the living and non-living matters.

AYURVEDA

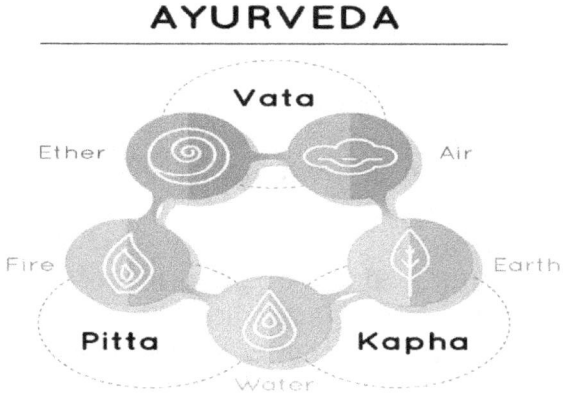

Practices done for a healthy living differ from person to person. This will depend on specific interactions among the five elements within the universe to form three unique life energies (the Vata, Pitta, and Kapha doshas). An individual possess all the three life energies, but only one will dominate over the remaining two. Every dosha has its own special effects on the body. They run the physiological processes of both the mind and body. The life energies are responsible for the special individual characteristics.

Specific Combinations of the Elements

All the substances involved will pair to form the three life forces. The Vata dosha (air and space), Pitta (fire and water) and the Kapha (earth and water). Depending on the life force that dominates in a person, his or her qualities will reflect the specific elemental characteristics in the combination.

The doshas proportions must match your birth makeup. If this is not the case, due to an imbalance in the doshic state, the person is considered unhealthy. The states of the doshas are usually described as follows:

- Balanced- when all the three life energies are available in their natural proportion.

- Depleted state- when a dosha is in a proportion less than the normal proportion.
- Aggravated state- occurs when the proportion of the dosha is more than the normal proportion.

Imbalance susceptibility is specific to the predominant dosha. This is one reason why Ayurveda, an individualized medication, is of importance. The intervention considers the life energy of a patient before considering any recovery procedure. The imbalances are detected before disease manifests. The Ayurvedic medicine is, therefore, more of a preventive rather than a curative process.

The Vata dosha.

The energy results after the natural combination of both the air and space. This is the driving force of both the Pitta and Kapha doshas. The life energy regulates the general body and mind movements. For this reason, Vata regulates all the body processes that involve movement. Scientists believe that the Vata is located within the bones, joints, ears, skin, colon as well as the nerve tissues.

The properties of the Vata include roughness, dryness, mobility, light and coldness. As a result, individuals with Vata as the predominant dosha are generally creative and with vitality. They are normally talkative, energetic, passionate, thinks fast and with a good communication skills.

Imbalance in the Vata

People with the predominant Vata are super active. An imbalance results in anxiety or fear. Due to their association with the body and mind movements, the Vatas, in the case of an aggregative effect will trigger raising of the adrenaline level responsible for the flight and fight responses. The reactions will lead to an increased heart beat rate, increased blood pressure, tightening of the muscles as well as the digestive system collapse.

Unresolved fear in the Vatas cascades both the nervous and endocrine systems. This will generate the states of general disquiet characterized with nail-biting habit, nervous habits and the inability to sit still. Bodily disorders like skin dryness and constipation are as well associated with the excessive state of the Vata proportion.

Some common practices associated with the imbalance.

Knowing your dominant dosha combination is important before considering the ayurvedic remedies available. Vata individuals have to avoid some habits considered unhealthy by the Ayurveda physicians. These include the following:

- Restrain from the use of stimulants like the alcohol, black coffee, and tea. Especially when they are cold.

- Eating foods are known to aggravate the Vata should be discouraged. These include the spicy foods.

- Avoid eating while feeling depressed or anxious.
- It is not advisable to eat while in a hurry. This might lead to the shutting down of the digestive system due to the pressure induced. Proper eating habit will give the digestive system time to perform the digestion process.

- The culture of going to bed late will lead to anxiety throughout the working hours. Enough sleep will give you enough rest. This will as a result balance the Vata dosha.

- Engaging in activities against your schedule can result in unnecessary pressure and hence the Vata imbalance. This is, therefore, not advisable for the Vatas.

Pitta Dosha

The Pitta dosha is a result of the combination of the water and fire elements. The dosha controls the energy production, metabolism as well as digestion. Some qualities of the Pitta life energy include the oily, light, hot, acidic, liquid, moving and sharp natures.

These characteristics reflect in the Pittas. The life force is located within the stomach, liver, pancreas, spleen, sweat glands and the blood channels. The physiological function of the Pitta dosha involves the breaking down of large food particles supplying the required energy and heat throughout the body.

Pitta individuals have a characteristic joy, courage, anger, jealousy, mental perception and willpower. The intelligent Pitters can engage in some actions that might lead to the life energy imbalance. Such actions replace the positive traits of the Pittas with the undesirable ones. The imbalance of this dosha manifests as inflammation, rashes, infection, heartburn or fever.

Considering actions that oppose the natural properties of the Pitta dosha will lead to its balance. For example, taking foods, supplements or even the therapeutic substances with different cooling properties to regulate the hot nature of the dosha will be of great help in balancing this life energy. Other useful interventions are illustrated below:

- It is advisable for the Pittas to avoid putting much pressure on themselves. Allowing yourself interval resting hours within the scheduled working hours will work well in balancing the Pitta dosha.

- Daily therapeutic massage to your body with cooling oils like the coconut oil will help in balancing the life energy.

- Engaging in activities that would calm the mind and body of the Pitta individuals are helpful in maintaining the dosha balance. A walk in the park will help you relax.

- Avoiding artificial stimulants like the cocaine is healthy. Such products will affect the natural Pitta composition making it imbalance.

- Regular intake of dairy products will help in maintaining the heat balance in Pitta.

Kapha dosha

This life energy results from the combination of both the earth and water. Ideally, when water and earth mix, mud is formed. Kapha is useful in governing the structure and stability in Kapha persons. Considering the properties, Kapha is heavy, static, soft, stable, slow, cool and oily. It is common for these features to reflect in Kapha individuals.

Kaphas have lubricated joints, bigger bones with a thick and oily skin. They also have a characteristic thick hair. They are always strong emotionally and physically. The additional strong immunity of the Kapha individual makes them more resistant to infections. Such individuals take time to make decisions. It is not easy to convince them otherwise once they decide on something. Loyalty to friends and partners is their principle.

Balancing the Kapha dosha for a healthy living

It is believed that anything movable, hot and light will oppose the original properties of the life energy. This will lead to the desired state of balance. Taking much focus on the Kapha calming diet like the foods that are light, dry, warm and rough is one intervention for maintaining the balance. Other Kapha pacifying actions include the following:

- One property of Kapha is that it is cold. Stimulation is, therefore, a calming intervention that will ensure the state of balance. Exposing the Kaphas to new experiences among other similar activities are some of the stimulating practices to enhance the state of dynamic.

- Kapha individuals are susceptible to cold and damp conditions. Kaphas normally complain of the congested respiratory system. Dry heat is used to ease the chest congestion. Neti pot, an Ayurvedic intervention, is also used in cleaning the respiratory tract preventing the undesirable congestion experiences.

- The other characteristic of the Kapha is their inactive nature. Engaging in physical activities like cycling and swimming will hinder the accumulation of harmful toxins within the body hence a healthy living.

- Stimulation of the general blood circulation is a Kapha balancing technique. This is done by a daily dry massage.

- Honey is said to facilitate the balancing of the Kapha. Other sweeteners, however, should be avoided since they increase the dosha leading to an imbalance. This might result in allergic reactions, sinuses, and lethargy. A tablespoon of unprocessed honey is, therefore, helpful in trimming off excess Kapha.

- Eating less food for dinner and allowing at least three hours for digestion before going to bed is a good virtue. The meal should consist of the food substances believed to facilitate the digestion drive within the body.

- Preferring the warm to cold foods and drinks promote balancing the Kapha. Intake of heated foods or those with natural heating properties like the spices is of great help. The warm particles are also easy to digest.

CHAPTER THREE: Dosha Online Test

Our bodies, emotions, behaviors and mental stability depend on the three life energies. These body types make a person different from the other since the combination of the five elements is unique in every individual. This means that people have individualized requirements to make them live a healthier and longer life. For instance, how we sleep, the food we eat and the exercises we engage in will not match the others preferences.

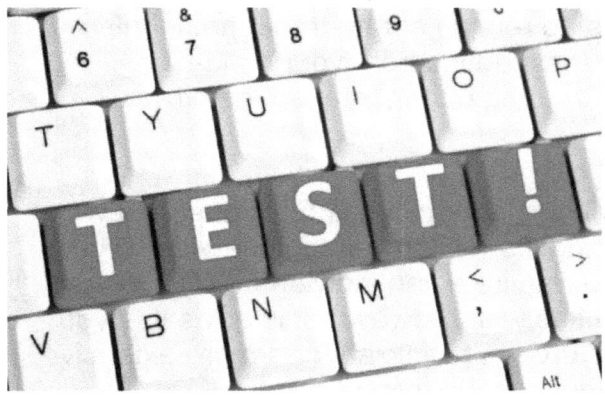

With these considerations, ayurvedic healthcare examines the unique body type of a patient before deciding on any recovery procedure. To live a promising life, you have to understand your dominant dosha combination. This will enable you to engage in activities that support your unique characteristics.

To help in managing your life appropriately, online dosha tests enable you to figure the proportions of all the three doshas in your body. With this, you can know your dominant life force. The outstanding force explains your distinctive mind-body structure. It is important to note that the life combinations are intrinsic. Online dosha tests involve two phases, the first set of the examination requires you to recall all your experiences when you were feeling happy and full of life.

The other phase of the test analyses the current state of your body to detect any change.
With the improved technology, you can identify your outstanding dosha combination and decide on the significant remedies for healthy living in case of an imbalance. Online diagnostic tests make it easy for any individual to remain strong throughout their lifetime. The tests define both your mind-body combination and the current state of health.

Diagnostic tests
Using the online platform is helpful in ensuring you live a promising life. This gives the overview of what practices you require as an individual to live longer and remain fit as well. However, it is advisable you consult an Ayurveda physician for a more extensive and professional dosha testing.
As mentioned above, a complex test clarifies both the dosha proportions as well as your current dosha state. Tests on the body types involve a series of steps to give comprehensive and useful feedbacks.

Determining the individual Prakriti
This test determines the balancing of all the three doshas in an individual. This will reflect the qualities and nature of a person making him or her different from the others. Prakriti explains the original body-mind composition. The test, therefore, entails remembering the quality life you lived when you were

feeling happy with full of life. The responses to questions in this phase of the test depend on the experiences during such times.

 It is not advisable to give feedbacks based on your current state. This is because they might be different due to various avoidable or unavoidable circumstances. Such answers, however, will be helpful in stage two of the examination. The questions have options and require you to choose the option that best describes your nature when in the correct state of health.
Some quizzes focus on the physical stature of the person undergoing the test. The hair texture and the color of the eye are some of the questions that require answers in this phase. In addition to the bodily traits, behavioral and psychological questions need honest answers for reliable outcomes.

The ultimate requirement of this analysis phase is to enable one understand their natural dosha composition. This, therefore, calls for honesty while providing responses to the questions. Consulting those close and understand you well will be a great advantage in providing answers that best define you. The approximated proportion of the tridosha is useful in determining both the dominant and secondary doshas. Performing the tests frequently, about three times a week will give your actual body-mind composition.

Determining the individual Vikruti
Knowing your Prakriti outcome will enable you to maximize on your potentials. Moreover, a Vikruti test will help you understand your current body type makeups for comparison with the Prakriti outcome.

When not in good health, the Vikruti results will not match your original dosha composition.

As a principle of the ayurvedic procedures, the root cause of a dosha imbalance has to be figured out before any intervention is implemented. When giving feedback to these questions, focus more on how you feel at the moment or a week earlier. The outcome will make you realize which of the dosha life energy is out of balance. This gives you the confidence in implementing an ayurvedic strategy that will reset the distorted equilibrium.

Repeating this test often is important in making sure you get a true picture of your mind-body composition. This will enable you to detect any change in the body type compositions for early intervention.

Dosha imbalance determination

The Prakriti and the Vikruti are compared to note any difference in the dosha compositions. The slightest change in dosha proportion basing on both the Prakriti and Vikruti tests will signify an imbalance. One dosha can influence the composition of the others and hence their states of balance. Further analysis of the two tests is very technical and requires a qualified ayurvedic medic to perform the operation. Since the Vata controls both the Pitta and Kapha doshas, ayurvedic physicians perform the Vata test first before concluding with the Kapha test.

Once the affected doshas are identified, the physician recommends a proven strategy to rectify the error. Vata proportion test is done ahead of the other two life energies since it is viewed as the driving force of the significant Pitta and Kapha forces. It is, therefore, the responsibility of the patient to follow the prescription by the ayurvedic practitioner as well as monitoring their recovering progress.

This is possible by regularly repeating the Vikrutis testing procedures when under the medication process. This notifies you in the case of positive progress.
After attaining the desired balance, it is good to follow all the requirements, as per the Ayurvedic professional, for a happy and healthy living depending on your predominant dosha combination.

CHAPTER FOUR: Herbal Remedies for Vata Dosha

Ayurvedic medicine limits the use of herbs as a primary strategy in correcting a condition whose root cause is clear as per the qualified ayurvedic practitioner. This medical approach views health as a favorable coordination between the mind and body for proper functioning. Vata is one dosha responsible for all the physiological movements of both the body and mind. This life force facilitates the other two Pitta and Kapha forces.

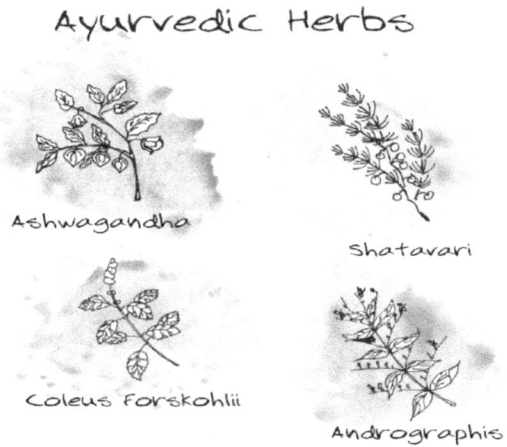

Ayurvedic Herbs

Ashwagandha

Shatavari

Coleus Forskohlii

Andrographis

Individuals with the predominant Vata energy are usually active and with vitality. Aggregative effects on the Vata would lead to anxiety and fear in persons with Vata as the predominant dosha. It is, therefore, necessary for the implementation of strategies that would balance the proportion of this dosha.

Qualified Ayurvedic medics utilize the herbs in rectifying the condition. As a principle of the Ayurveda, the remedy does not control the symptoms of ill health but manages the ultimate cause. Herbal remedies for the Vata dosha are available and useful under prescription by a professional to bring back the lost state of equilibrium.

The proven Vata dosha pacifying herbs

The Ayurveda applies the principle of `opposite' to calm all the doshas and attain their state of balance. In the case of imbalance, the heavy, sweet, calming and warming herbs are helpful to counter the dry, light, cold as well as the mobility natures of the Vata life energy. Before choosing the best herb to pacify your imbalanced Vata, it is important you identify the specific point from where the Vata imbalance is triggered.

Vidari

This herb is helpful in maintaining the mind-body coordination for healthy living. Vidari is a long time Vata pacifying agent. It was also ideal for promoting the reproductive system of an individual. For example, its spermatogenic property is helpful in the production of sperms in men.

The heart beat rate of persons with imbalanced Vata dosha rises to abnormal rate. This tuber contains the cardio-tonic property to restore the normal health of the heart.

Infections of the alimentary canal reveal by vomiting of the infected. This occurs after the aggregation of the Vata life force. The antiemetic nature of this herb helps in leveling the dosha composition to a state of dynamic hence treating the real cause of the adverse vomiting. The tuber minimizes the dryness of the intestine thereby reducing constipation experienced by the affected in case of a loss in Vata balance.

Increased blood pressure is also a sign that the Vata life force is out of balance. The *Pueraria tuberrosa* features a hypotensive property that lowers the pressure to the desired level. The Ayurvedic medicine also clears the throat to assist in the management of coughs.

Adverse effects of the Vidari herb
The therapeutic consumption of this herb is limited to prescription by a professional ayurvedic medic. This is because it has adverse side effects to the lovers:

- Its contraceptive nature hinders the development of ovum in women. It is, therefore, not recommended for pregnant women unless under the prescription of an ayurvedic physician.

- Infertility in women who carelessly use the root tuber is on the rise. This is because of the anti-implantation property of the vidari plant. The abortifacient nature of this herb has the ability to terminate a developing fetus. The plant is, thus, associated with miscarriages.

- Due to its ability to hinder the biological effects of the male eggs, the uncontrolled use of the herb will lead to male infertility.

Ashwagandha

This is one of the most powerful herbal remedies in case of an imbalance of the mind-body functioning. This shrub belongs to the same class as the tomato. The shrub has some important therapeutic properties. As an adaptogenic substance, this shrub manages your response to both the internal and external stresses.

The presence of the anticonvulsant characteristic in this plant has made it applicable in preventing seizure that might lead to harmful physical convulsion. This enhances the mental health of an individual. In addition to this, the herb acts as an anti-depressant.

This shrub has some antibacterial properties that control infections caused by the bacteria. As an ayurvedic remedy, this property maintains the health of the gut as well as the respiratory tract by countering the actions of the bacteria. It also protects the urinogenital.
The botanic regulates the blood sugar level. Ashwagandha controls the diabetic condition associated with the abnormal sugar level.

Health issues of this herbal remedy

- Large doses of the ashwagandha can induce abortion. This is one reason as to why consultation of the qualified ayurvedic practitioner is helpful before you consume the shrub for its therapeutic characteristics.

- Ashwagandha can interact with other medications especially the anti-depressant drugs. Consider the instructions of a medical personnel dealing with the Ayurveda to avoid such harmful interactions.

- Uncontrolled consumption of this herb can affect the alimentary canal leading to gastrointestinal conditions like diarrhea and nausea.

Bala

Bala is an ancient ayurvedic medicine that was anciently appropriate in enhancing the skeletal strength. According to the Ayurveda policy, the Vata dosha is located within the joints hence the need to use this herb as a remedy in case of the dosha magnification in these sites.

The roots of this plant contain the beta-sitosteols with the immune-modulatory properties. This regulates the functions of the immune system to ensure it functions sufficiently.

This herb also assists in digestion by enhancing expiration of harmful substances from the body. Toxic gasses might be produced during the breaking down of foods. The digestion issues can worsen due to an imbalance of the Vata dosha.

Vata dosha is distributed at the joints. Upon aggravation of this life force, the wear and tear of these joints occur. This is characterized by a lot of pain and inflammation at these sites. The Bala has the ability to retain the Vata balance.

Side effects of the Bala as a Vata pacifier

- The herb contains the minimal composition of ephedrine that is to some extent responsible in aggravation the Vata body type. This results in heart attack, high blood pressure among other effects of the imbalanced dosha. There is no scientific proof to confirm this statement.

- The use of this herb has to be regulated based on the instruction of the ayurvedic physician. This herbal medication is functional in children and during lactation but not recommended for the pregnant mothers.

CHAPTER FIVE: Herbal Remedies for Pitta Dosha

Fire and water naturally combine to form the Pitta life energy. The force is responsible for the transformative functions of both the body and mind. An imbalance can either occur due to increase or decrease in the normal proportion of the dosha. Aggravated level of this Pitta energy manifests as heartburn, bitter taste in the mouth, skin rashes and fever. On the other hand, too little Pitta will aggravate the levels of the other Vata and Kapha body types. This leads to poor digestion and emotional imbalance.

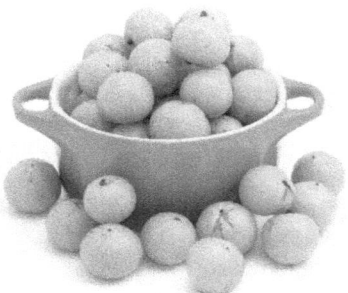

1- Amalaki (also known as Indian Gooseberry)

Pacifying the out of balance Pitta dosha is vital in ensuring a healthy livelihood. So many Ayurvedic interventions have been useful for the past years. The use of natural herbs as an ayurvedic medication has proven to be of great significance. The properties of such plants enable them to be first choice herbal remedies when it comes to balancing the Pitta life force.

Pitta pacifying herbs for a healthy living
Shatavari

This Shatavari herb has long been used to promote the reproductive health in women hence the name "a woman with 100 husbands." The nourishing properties of this plant help in controlling certain conditions believed to result from poor coordination of both the body and mind compositions due to overheating.

As an Ayurvedic medicine, this herb controls the balance of the Pitta life energy. This plant has cooling and soothing effects that manage conditions resulting from imbalanced Pitta energy. The combined sweet and bitter taste of safari plant will counter the normal properties of the overheated Pitta, thereby, maintaining the correct state of dynamic. Fortunately, this agent is also known to balance the Vata life force in case it is triggered.

The immunomodulation property of this botanical promotes the functions of macrophages and hence strengthening the immune system of persons against infections. According to the Ayurvedic medics, infection within the body occurs because of a Pitta imbalance. This property of the plant, therefore, facilitates balancing of the life energy for maximum protection against external stressors.

The combined grounding and nourishing features of this useful product promote the functioning of the digestive organs resulting from loss of symmetry in the Pitta energy. This plant treats the gastrointestinal

malfunctioning that might occur from an improper body-mind coordination.
Sexual functionality depends on the mind-body harmonization.

This plant helps in the treatment of sexual debility in both the male and female. The strategy rejuvenates the loss of libido in males. Undesirable pH readings of the vaginal walls might lead to loss of sexual interest as well. This plant, therefore, cleans the reproductive organs to maintain the state of dynamic for maximum sexual fun.

Pitta imbalance is evident as an irritation of the respiratory membrane. The irritation occurs when the respiratory tract becomes dry after the interference of the dosha proportion. Shatavari herb harmonizes this effect hence controlling the bronchitis fever. This is because the botanical balances all the body fluids moisturizing the breathing system in the process.

Negative effects of using Shatavari herb
Individuals who are allergic to asparagus should not use the herb as an ayurvedic remedy. This might lead to the skin conditions as well as pulmonary malfunctions.
Uncontrolled usage of this herb is linked to abnormal weight gain. The usage of this plant as a medication should follow a directive by a qualified Ayurvedic practitioner.
The exact contraindication of the phytoestrogens in this herb is unclear. Those with estrogen sensitivity are advised to avoid substances with phytoestrogen.

Neem

Neem is applied as an ayurvedic agent because of its bitter and cooling nature. The herb can balance both the Pitta and Kapha doshas. It was originally used as a strategy for a quality skin condition. The balance of the Pitta is achieved by removing the excess.

Ayurveda connects the health of our hair with that of the bones. They believe that hair problems occur when the mind-body operations are altered. Imbalances in the three doshas affect the quality and therefore important to understand your dominant dosha combination. Pitta imbalance manifests as gray hair. Neem cleanses the blood acting as a natural agent against dandruff that affects the hair quality.

The calming nature of the neem calls for the topical application of the neem to treat the skin conditions. The health of the skin depends on the cleanliness of the blood. Contaminated blood manifests as boils on the skin. Neem detoxifies the blood hence reducing the Pitta concentration. This leads to a balancing of the life force, thus, enhancing the skin health.

Ideally, hypertension result from liver malfunctioning as well as excessive internal heat. For the Ayurvedic application of neem, this condition is linked with an imbalanced Pitta. The cooling nature of these leaves helps in regulating the accumulated heat responsible for the chronic disease. This property of the neem is also important in preventing sudden heart attacks by regulating the accumulation of fat around the heart.

Undermining factors for the use of neem as an ayurvedic medicine.

The bitter nature of neem makes it revolting. It is because of this that most Ayurvedic medics advise their clients to mix it with other sweet and healthy substances like the honey.

Uncontrolled application of this herb might lead to aggravation of the Vata causing secondary health effects. Pregnant women are not advised to take the plant for the medical purpose since it can result in extreme fatigue if abused.

Neem products for external uses contains some carriers that when ingested can lead to toxication of the body. It, therefore, not advisable to store it where a child can access it easily.

Amalaki

The Indian gooseberry was originally the best in protecting the users against skin conditions, diabetes, lung conditions among other chronic conditions resulting from the dosha imbalance. The contents of this fruit have ayurvedic properties that ensure balance in all the three life energies. Ayurveda links all the health conditions with the balance between the body and mind constituents.

Because of the natural vitamin C contained in this herb, Amla helps in reducing the concentration of the Pitta dosha without affecting the concentration of either the Vata and Kapha life energies.

Excessive heat within the digestive tract indicates an imbalance of the Pitta dosha due to its aggravation. The cooling effect of this botanical removes the excess Pitta composition from within the alimentary canal. This ensures a smooth stomach lining with all the constituents working to their maximum. This illustrates that this herb balances the digestive fire.

Natural toxins in the body system affect the mind-body operations. This is because of the increased concentration of the Pitta concentration. The Amla has the property of detoxifying the tissues and in the process cleaning the bowels for maximum functioning.
Excess concentration of the Pitta dosha at the joints might lead to inflammation. This is characterized by pain that makes the affected individuals uneasy. The Amla has a cooling characteristic that is utilized in soothing the affected site. The presence of vitamin C in this herb improves the overall immune system of the user.

As an Ayurvedic medicine, Amalaki breaks down cholesterol to healthy levels, thereby, enhancing the health of the heart. Also, it stimulates the production of Ojas that maintains the blood sugar level in case of a Pitta imbalance.

Side effects of using the Amalaki as an ayurvedic medicine
Individuals with iron deficiencies should avoid using the Amla. This is because it forms chelates with iron and in the process reduce the iron counts within the blood for use by the body.
Pittas suffering from gastrointestinal conditions like diarrhea must not use this fruit as an ayurvedic remedy since it can worsen the condition.

Taking the herb at night should be discouraged since it erodes the enamel. This leads to dental conditions like the weakening of the affected teeth. Excessive dosage of this fruit can also weaken the dental formulae and should, therefore, be controlled.

CHAPTER SIX: Herbal Remedies for Kapha Dosha

Like the other two doshas, a balanced Kapha supports the mind-body coordination for healthy living. This energy life forms when the water and earth naturally combines. The main function of this life force is stabilizing the body structure and physiology.

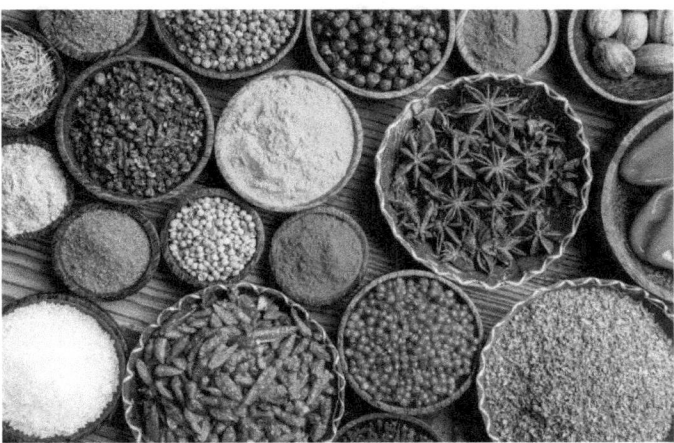

2-Selection of Spices Including Turmeric

An imbalance in the Kapha dosha occurs when the concentration within the body shoots to an abnormal level. This manifest in many forms. For example, one feels depressed, lazy and feels sleepy after taking a meal. Signs of the Kapha imbalance are not limited to those mentioned above.

Treatment for the loss of equilibrium within the system is important for a fruitful and longer life. Elimination of the primary cause is the best remedy to help in regaining the lost balance. It is, therefore, important to identify the undesirable practices and foods that increase the concentration of the Kapha life force.

Ayurvedic physicians relate all the health conditions with the balance of the tridosha. They believe that to rectify the uncommon state, they have to identify the predominant dosha of their patients. Health interventions are recommended to counter the adverse effects, thereby, regaining the original body-mind physiological functions. Herbs have since been helpful in maintaining the states of balance in all the important life energies.

The common Kapha pacifying herbs
Many herbs help in maintaining the balance of the Kapha body type. The unique characteristics of these plants give them the importance in achieving the desired balance.

Kalmegha
Andrographis paniculate is a traditional plant that was used as a medicine to manage fever as well as jaundice. They grow naturally in the tropical and subtropics. The therapeutic features of this plant made the Ayurvedic practitioners gain interest in its use in leveling the dosha balance for a healthy body-mind coordination.

Most of the natural sweeteners aggravate the Kapha concentration of an individual leading to an imbalance. The bitter kalmegh regulates the sweet nature of this life energy balancing the life energy. Because of this nature, the herb is applicable in managing the diabetic conditions in persons with a predominant Kapha body type. The bitter leaves can also wash the stomach to enhance quality functioning and a balanced state of dynamic.

The tonic property of this plant provides additional strength to the body. The Kaphas are usually strong by nature. In the case of an imbalance of the Kapha life energy, the individuals become weaker. This botanical is useful in promoting the automated body-mind coordination after the achievement of the lost state of balance.

The oily nature of the Kapha dosha makes the individuals with this predominant life energy have a smooth and healthy skin. In the case of imbalance, the skin becomes dry and unattractive. Contaminated blood manifests as a boil or the patches. This plant has a blood purifying property that detoxifies the blood making it clean. In this way, the Kapha dosha is balanced.

Kaphas are characterized with strong immunity against infections. Eating foods that raise the Kapha concentration will eventually weaken the immune functioning. This herb has an antipyretic nature that acts against diarrheal infections of the alimentary canal.

Side effects of using kalmegh as an herbal remedy for Kapha dosha

This herb has an anti-fertility feature that makes it not advisable for the pregnant mothers. Uncontrolled use of this plant can also lead to sterility of both men and women abusing its usage.

This herb is linked to duodenal ulcers and bleeding disorders if its usage is not controlled. Consultation of a professional Ayurvedic practitioner should be necessary to understand your health conditions before any herbal intervention to balance your dosha composition.

Turmeric
From the past, turmeric has been included in the diet as a supplement. This is because of its health importance to the users. Its application in the Ayurveda was because of its ability to facilitate the body-mind functioning. The unique characteristics of this plant make it helpful in maintaining the balances of the available life energies.

People with the Kapha as the predominant dosha have a strong immunity against infections. An imbalance of this life energy kills the immune cells responsible for protection against diseases. Turmeric has an antioxidant property that promotes the working of the immune cells against infections.

In the case of imbalance, the digestion process fails. As an Ayurvedic medicine, turmeric has the property of promoting protein digestion. This maintains the standard body-mind functioning.
The cold nature of Kapha can be worsened during winter to an abnormal level rendering the life energy imbalance. The bitter taste of this herb ensures the achievement of the desired state of equilibrium. The taste will produce heat within the body to regulate the excess cold experienced by the affected Kaphas.

Turmeric contains natural blood purifiers. These components remove the toxins that contaminate the blood. These toxicants might lead to heart failure if not controlled early. With turmeric, the heart and general circulatory system are safe from infections. The safety is due to the body's state of equilibrium.

Kaphas are considered strongest of all the tridosha. Excessive accumulation of this life energy will mean the dosha is out of balance. The Kaphas, on the contrary, becomes weaker than normal. The Ayurvedic turmeric is believed to provide the Divine Mother's energy according to the users.

Contraindications of using turmeric as an ayurvedic medicine

Excessive usage of this herb during pregnancy might lead to complications. Consult your ayurvedic medic on the amount of turmeric to add into your normal diet when heavy with a child. Those people under medication aimed at inhibiting the unnecessary production of blood platelets should avoid using this ayurvedic herb for whatever reason.

Pippali

Pippali is an ayurvedic herb that grows in warm regions. The herb is commonly helpful in managing a number of disorders without taking into consideration the balance of the life energies. Ayurvedic medics utilize the ability of this plant in balancing the tridosha to boost the quality of life. This takes advantage of the various outstanding properties of this botanic.

This remedy is mostly important during the spring season. The plant has the ability to restore the lungs in the case of a Kapha dosha imbalance. During this period, the individual with Kapha as the predominant body type is exposed to allergens among other infectious agents. This herb liquefies mucus within the breathing system to help in regaining the lost balance.

Loss of the Kapha balance leads to Manda Agni. This means that the body does not perform its functions to the maximum. Pippali has the ability to ignite the digestive fire in case of any gastric infection or dysfunction. This facilitates the absorption of nutrients and elimination of contaminants from the body.

Unlike other herbs, pippali is tridoshic. It has the ability to harmonize all the body types. This makes it capable of supporting a greater number of functions. For example, this herb can solve all the digestive abnormalities. This is because the remedy has the ability to cool the out of balance Pitta dosha due to its cooling property.

Issues associated with the use of Pippali

The users should, not abuse Pippali since it is a very powerful herb. Over-dosing this substance will prove to be harmful to your overall body-mind functioning.

CHAPTER SEVEN: Delicious Dosha Recipes

According to Ayurveda, people have unique body-mind setups. The five elements of the universe systematically pair to form the tridosha. Every individual has all the three life energies, but only one is dominant over the others. This brings about the unique characteristics of a person.

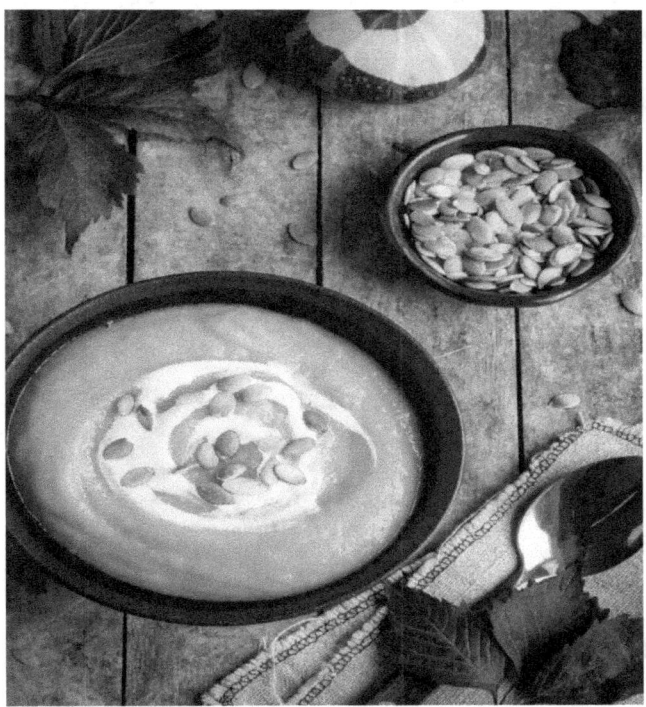

Maintaining the balance of these doshas is vital for the individual wellbeing. It is important to identify your predominant life force in order to live a healthy and productive life. How we live and feed will either maintain the doshas' states of equilibrium or lose their balance.

Each of the three life forces has outstanding properties. Depending on the predominant life force, different recipes work for different people. Visiting your Ayurvedic physician is, therefore, important before changing your normal diet.

Important recipes for a balanced Vata dosha

Opting for the diets with qualities counteracting those of the Vata. The warm, moist, stabilizing and grounding foods will ensure balancing of the Vata in case of an imbalance.

The sweet curried pumpkin soup

This recipe provides balance to the Vata. Pumpkin has some moist characteristics that maintain the Vata equilibrium. Spices are added to meet the Vatas' tastes.

Ingredients
- 2 sugar pumpkins for roasting
- ½ teaspoon cinnamon
- 2 tablespoon of ghee
- 2 cups of coconut milk
- Salt
- ½ cup sliced Vidalia onion

Preparation procedure
Customize pumpkin wells by cutting them into halves and removing the seeds. Introduce sprinkles of the ghee, coconut milk, a pinch of salt and the cinnamon. Out of the modified well, produce other two shafts then add the sliced Vidalia onions and an extra

cinnamon before placing it in a preheated oven for about 40 minutes to roast.

The roasted food is allowed to cool before scooping the soft flesh with the ingredients added to it. Blend the scooped product while adding more milk into the pitcher during the process. Adding salt to the final recipe will make it palatable.

Gingered carrots

This recipe takes into account the Ayurvedic properties of the carrot, ghee, Organic Vata Churna and ginger to produce maximum dosha balance.

Ingredient
- 2 cups of Julienned carrots
- 2 tablespoon of fresh grated ginger roots
- Salt
- ½ teaspoon Organic Vata Churna
- 2 tablespoons brown sugar
- 1 tablespoon ghee

Preparation procedure
For three minutes, boil the carrots in water containing the Organic Vata Churna. After the time limit expires, remove the carrot from the oven.
In a different frying sheet, heat ghee while adding ginger and brown sugar on it. Allow the cocktail to heat for the next three minutes.

To the pan containing heated ghee, add the already heated carrot and allow them to cook for the next five minutes or so. Add a little salt to make it appetizing. Serve the food while warm to counter the cold nature of the Vata. This will produce quantity enough to sustain two people.

Lemon Rice

The sour taste of lemon allows the balance of the Vata constituents. Adding it to your diet provides greater health benefits. Enough to serve two people, the following quantities of ingredients are required.

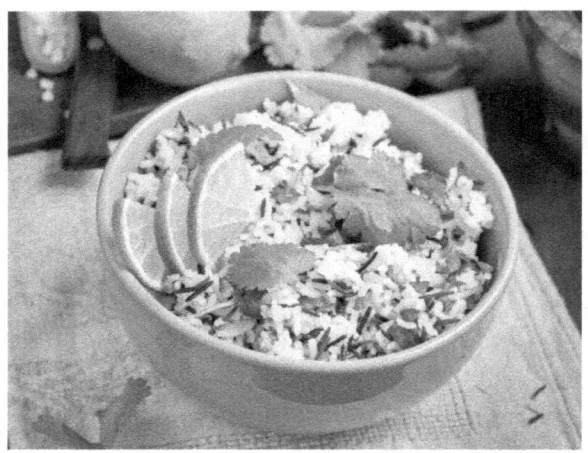

Ingredients
- ¾ cup basmati rice
- 1½ cups Water
- 2 teaspoon seeds ghee
- ¼ teaspoon of Turmeric
- 1 teaspoon black mustard
- ½ cup of Fresh lemon juice
- ¼ tablespoon Salt

Recipe preparations

After washing basmati rice to remove any contaminants, boil it in water for about 20-30 minutes then remove the cover to allow evaporation to take place till the rice finish cooking.

Heat the mustard seeds in ghee until they begin to pop. Remove the seeds from the oven and allow it to be cool. Add turmeric, salt and the lemon juice to the cooled seeds to make it desirable.

The spice combination is then added to the already cooked rice and mixed well. Serve the food while it is still warm.

Curried Tofu and Dinosaur Kale

Ingredients
- ➢ 3 cups of chopped dinosaur Kale
- ➢ ¼ cup toasted sunflower seeds
- ➢ 2 thinly sliced shallots
- ➢ 1 package of drained firm organic tofu
- ➢ 2 teaspoons of curry powder
- ➢ ½ tablespoon of ghee
- ➢ Lemon juice with 50% lemon content
- ➢ 2 tablespoons virgin olive oil
- ➢ Salt

Recipe preparation
Over medium temperature, heat ½-tablespoon ghee then adds ¼-cup sunflower seeds. Remove the pan from the oven once the seeds turn golden brown. Over the same medium hotness, heat the 2 tablespoons of the olive oil. Add the thinly sliced shallots together with the curry powder. Leave it in the oven until the shallots become translucent. Tofu is included into the mixture then stirred to cover the tofu with curry. The tofu is allowed to turn brown while on the pan for about 8 minutes.

Within these 8 minutes, add the already chopped Sukuma wiki on the tofu. Squeeze lemon and salt on

top of the mixture while continuing to stir until the kale stalk cook.
The toasted sunflower seeds are spread over the already served dish.

Important recipes for a balanced Pitta dosha
Considering the hot nature of the Pitta dosha, for example, a cool and nourishing recipe will maintain the wonderful body-mind coordination.

Coconut rice
Ingredients
- ➢ 1 cup of basmati rice
- ➢ 2 tablespoon of coconut oil
- ➢ 3 cups of water
- ➢ salt
- ➢ 3 cups of water
- ➢ ½-cup coconut flakes

Preparation
Boil 3 cups of water before adding the rice, coconut oil, and the coconut flakes. Reduce the amount of heat then cover the rice to cook well. For the balancing of Pitta dosha, avoid much salt since it is linked to the aggravation of the dosha.
 The remaining coconut flake is turned to brown by roasting. This done while waiting for the rice to be ready.

The roasted flakes are spread over the cooked rice as a sauce when serving. Basmati is served while still warm and tender.

Asparagus Saffron Risotto with Lemon

Ingredients

- ➤ 2 tablespoon of ghee
- ➤ ¼ whole lemon
- ➤ 1 cup of risotto
- ➤ 2 cups of asparagus
- ➤ ¼ teaspoon of black paper
- ➤ 1 teaspoon of cumin
- ➤ ½ teaspoon of salt
- ➤ 2 pinch of Saffron
- ➤ Enough water

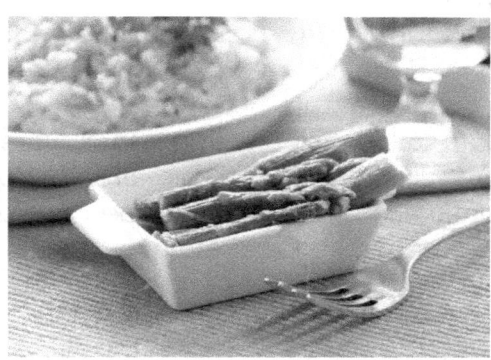

Preparation of the recipe

Manually grind the saffron while adding water to dissolve it completely. Allow it to rest for about 10 minutes. In the meantime, clean and cut into cubes the asparagus.

In a pot containing ghee, fry the cumin seeds then add the diced asparagus, risotto and other ingredients like the black pepper before the seeds turn brown. Fry further for an additional ½-a minute before adding a cup of boiling water. Add a cup of water after every five minutes until the meal is ready.

Roasted Coconut Sesame Oatmeal

Ingredients

- ➢ 1 cup of oats
- ➢ 1 teaspoon of coconut oil
- ➢ 3 tablespoons of coconut flakes
- ➢ 3 cups of water
- ➢ 3 tablespoon of sesame seeds
- ➢ 1 teaspoon of raw sugar

Recipe preparation

Boil 2 cups of water then reduce the heat before adding oil and sugar. Allow the mixture to boil further. In the meantime, use a coffee grinder to grind the oat to smaller particles.

Under controlled temperature, dry roast both the sesame seeds and the coconut flakes while frequently stirring to prevent them from burning.

The ground oatmeal is mixed with a cup of water. Salt is added before mixing them with the already boiling water. Cook until all the water is absorbed and the food becomes creamy, soft and even.

Serve the meal with toasted sesame seeds and coconut flakes.

Almond Date Shake with Cinnamon

Ingredients

- ➢ 2 whole dried dates
- ➢ 1/8 inch ginger
- ➢ 1 cup of almond milk
- ➢ 2 pinch of cinnamon

Recipe preparation

Crush all the three ingredients in a blender. This should be served at room temperature.

Acorn Squash with Ghee & Maple Syrup

Ingredients

- ➢ 1 acorn squash
- ➢ 1 tablespoon of maple syrup
- ➢ ¼ teaspoon of salt
- ➢ 1 tablespoon of ghee

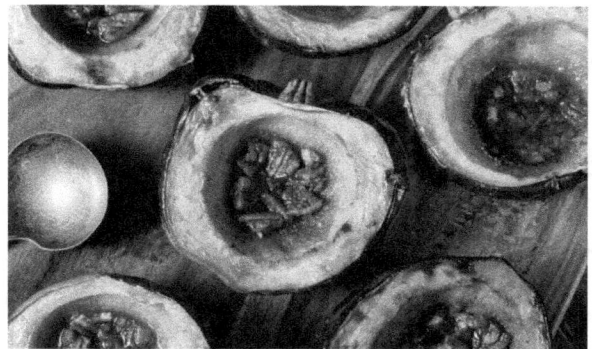

3-Homemade Roasted Acorn Squash

Recipe preparation
Cut the whole acorn squash into halves. Place one-half in the 8x8-casserole dish then drizzle the maple syrup, ghee and the salt.
Poking of the acorn is necessary to allow the flavor to be absorbed into the acorn. Bake it for one hour while covered before serving.

Important recipes for a balanced Kapha dosha
Too much of Kapha constitution lead to the Kapha imbalance condition among the Kaphas. Recipes that are warm, dry, light and with moderated amount of salt harmonizes the concentration of this life force facilitating a well-coordinated body-mind relationship. The properties counter the cool, moist and heavy nature of the Kapha.

Chickpea with Coconut Pesto
Ingredients

- ➢ 1 tablespoon of olive oil
- ➢ ½ cup of coconut milk

- ¼ teaspoon of salt
- ½ whole lime
- ½ a cup of basil
- 2 pinch cayenne pepper
- 1-cup chickpea

Recipe preparation

Whisk all the coconut milk, olive oil and the lime juice to produce a homogenous product. Pound all the coconut base chopped basil and salt in a food processor for uniformity. Set aside the paste to enhance its flavors.

Light-fry the chickpeas in a frying pan with sprinkled olive oil until the chickpeas turns slightly brown and crunchy.

Mix both the sauce and the chickpeas in a pan before serving it with little garnish of basil on top and a slice of lemon.

Ginger Basil Limeade
Ingredients

- 2 teaspoons of raw sugar
- 1 whole lime
- ½ cup of basil
- 2 inch of fresh ginger

Recipe preparation

With the help of a fine grater, shave the skin of the whole lime into a lime zest. Chop the ginger into pieces and then juice the lime.

Into a blender containing the lime juice, lime zest, a handful of basil leaves and raw sugar add one cup of water and turn on the machine. The final blend will be smooth and uniform.

Add three cups of water to the ginger-lime juice still in the blender pitcher. Chill and serve it with fresh basil as the sauce.

Salting the rim of your drinking glass will ensure you benefit from all the six tastes for a balanced body-mind operation.

Almond Milk Chai
Ingredients
- ➢ 1 tablespoon of maple syrup
- ➢ ¼ inch of fresh ginger
- ➢ 2 pinch nutmeg
- ➢ 1 cup of almond milk
- ➢ ¼-teaspoon cinnamon
- ➢ 2 teaspoon of ghee
- ➢ ¼-teaspoon of cardamom

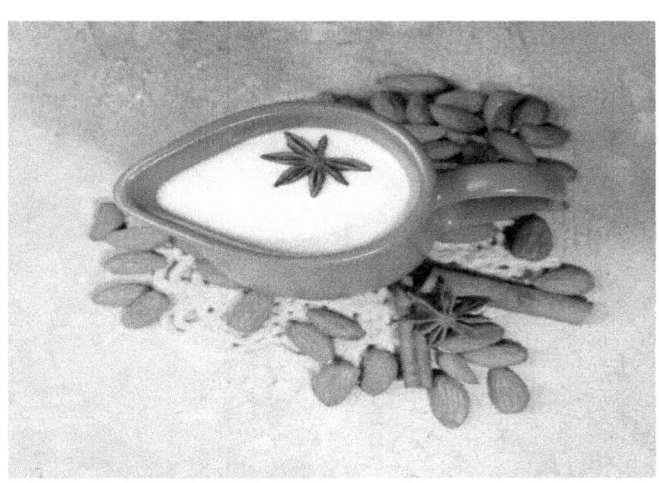

Recipe preparation

Watch the almond milk as it boils to prevent it from overflowing during the steaming process. After it starts to simmer, turn off the heat then add the other ingredients to spice it up. Brew the final product for about five minutes before serving.

CONCLUSION

Health is not merely the absence of disease. The coordination of the mind, body and spirit will define your wellbeing.
The five elements (fire, earth, water, space and air) of the universe systematically pair with each other to form three life energies: the Vata (air and space), Pitta (fire and water) and the Kapha (water and earth).

These inherent life forces, according to Ayurvedic practitioners, determine the quality of life. Every person has the tridosha with only one dosha dominant over the remaining two. The dominant body type makes a person different from the others.

An imbalance in any of the three doshas signifies poor health. It is, therefore, important for every person to analyze him or herself to identify his or her predominant life force. The online platform provides quizzes that when given honest responses, can reflect your true dosha compositions. Though this gives the overview on how you should live to sustain your unique body type, consulting a professional is vital for the reliable outcome and the best corrective strategies.
To maintain a balanced body-mind functioning, enjoy the different recipes that have the capability of neutralizing the state of all the three life energies. Ensure that you consume foods and spices that are beneficial for your specific body types.

In the case of an imbalance of any of the three doshas, consult a qualified ayurvedic medic on the best herbs to help manage the off balance. These plants have properties that counter the original qualities of the life forces suppose an imbalance occurs.

Determine your predominant dosha and choose the foods that will help in maintaining your health. Turn to the therapeutic nature of the botanic to ensure your spirit, body and mind are harmonized.

The Definitive Guide of Intermittent Fasting

How to Benefit from Fasting and is it for Everyone

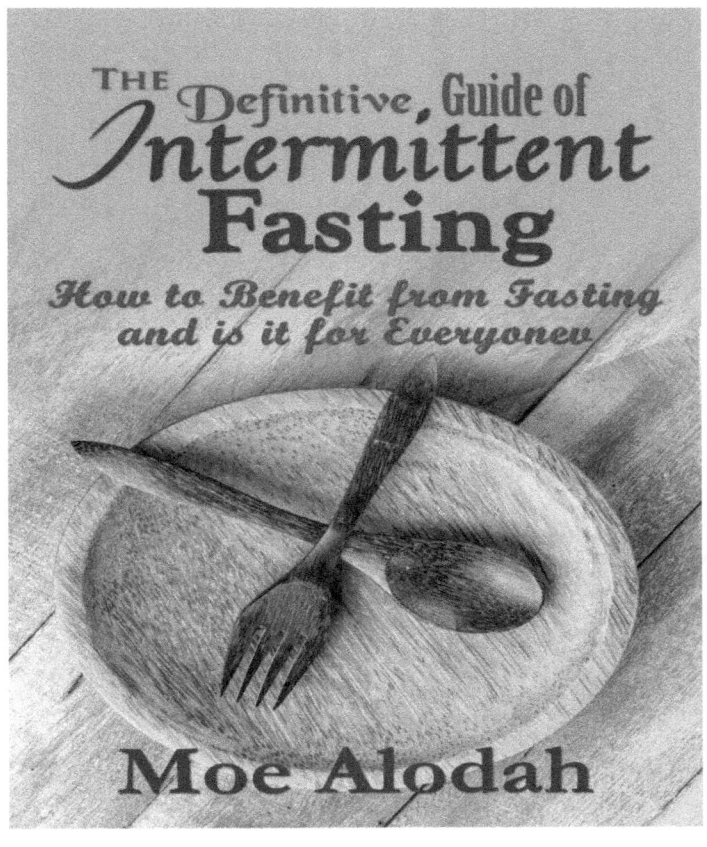

TABLE OF CONTENTS

Bonus Chapter

CHAPTER ONE: What is Intermittent Fasting (IF)?

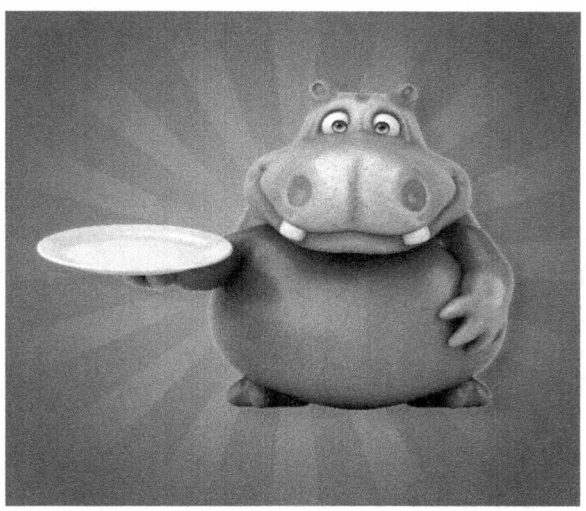

Excess foods are stored within the body either as glycogen or as fat for future use. The body requires time, therefore, to utilize them. For example, during the night when you sleep, you are in a state where your body utilizes the stored nutrients during the fasting period to maintain the normal body functioning.

This is the fasting period. The first meal we take when we wake tends to break your fast and hence the name breakfast. In addition to this, our bodies undergo states of fasting where they break down the foods to produce the necessary energy every time we are not eating. Because of this, it is now important to note that fasting is part of our daily life.

Unlike starvation, which involves the involuntary absence of food, fasting is the intentional withholding of foods for either health or spiritual among others reasons best known to the practitioners. This, therefore, means that one can decide when to start a fast as well as stopping it. The eating pattern that recycles between the fasting and feasting is what is now known as intermittent fasting. It focuses on when to eat rather than what to eat.

The main aim of fasting is to allow the body use the stored energy. With this in mind, it is important to avoid foods rich in calories. However, taking coffee, tea, and water among other non-caloric beverages is advisable when you are in the starvation mode. Due to the many forms of fasting, some types allow the intake of low-calorie foods. The different forms are explained in detail later in the book. During this hunger period, supplements are important provided there are no calories in them. This reenergizes the body. The water prevents the body against dehydration. Lack of enough nutrients in our diet would call for the substitution.

How intermittent fasting operates

It is important first to note that life is all about the balance. For example, a balance between the yin and the yang as well as the balance between the good and the bad. This also applies to eating and fasting. During this fasting, the body utilizes its own fats (the excess fat) to produce energy.

When we eat, our bodies use the energy they require and the excess stored for later use. This is dictated by the presence of the insulin hormone. The increase in the level of insulin during the eating process facilitates the body to store the excess energy by linking it to the long-chain glycogen and then storing them in the liver. Due to the limited space in the liver, some sugar is converted to fat through a process called lipogenesis.

On the other hand, when we are not eating, the insulin within the body decreases and hence signals the body to begin burning the stored energy because the blood glucose level falls during this time.

The easily accessible source of energy during a fast is the glycogen. The compound is broken down into glucose molecules to facilitate the functioning of the body cells. Study indicate that the energy from breaking down glycogen is only capable of driving the body system for about 24-36 hours before the body begins to act on the stored fat as the ultimate source of energy.

It can now be deducted that for healthy living, a state of balance between the fasting and feasting periods is vital. Throughout our lives, it is either we are storing the food or breaking them down. This will mean that there is no weight net gain. Eating from the time we wake up until we go to sleep would lead to the addition of weight since the body acts on the food and further stores the excess. Opting to fast would avert this since more time would be available to burn the stored fat. This should not be an issue since our bodies are designed to work that way.

Factors that hinder one from considering the intermittent fasting.

The evidence-based benefits of intermittent fasting have triggered many to try it for healthy living.

However, many factors prevent people from trying this healthy intervention.

A. The fear of being hungry

Regardless of the benefits that come along with intermittent fasting, the body takes much time to adapt and hence the individual. Most people avoid this ancient program because they hate the feeling of being hungry and the discomfort that comes along with the feeling. However, with time your body would have better control over your hunger.

B. Desire for an immediate impact

It is always said that the emotionally strong personalities have patience and optimism in whatever program they engage in. With the belief that this fasting would help you have control over your weight, it is good to remain focused on the diet patterns.

However, the positive effects take much time to manifest (usually three weeks). Most people feel discouraged because of this and end up giving up on it. For example, losing weight with intermittent fasting should not be seen as a race but as the best alternative ever.

C. Fear of losing muscles

Regarding the study by many companies, it is believed that failing to take about 30g of protein after every few hours forces our body to break the muscles as the source of energy.

On the contrary, our bodies are adapted to preserving the muscles even while we are fasting. Again, there is no difference to the body between the proteins taken in a shorter period compared to protein spread throughout the day. This is because protein takes much time before absorption by the body.

In short, it is important to give this program a shot and experience how effectively you would lose weight among other health benefits associated with the program.

Important tricks for effective fasting

- **Never freak out**

It is obvious to be nervous when trying something new. You will ask yourself several rhetorical questions making you eventually change your mind about trying a new idea. This should not be the case when you need to enjoy the health benefits that come with intermittent fasting.

Our body act like a machine and would eventually adapt to the new dieting pattern. Pilon once advised that we should view fasting as a break from eating rather than a period of deficiency.

- **Always stay busy**

It is always said that an idle mind is the devil's workshop. Sitting around thinking about how hungry you are would tempt you into stopping your fast. Engage in activities that would keep you busy to scavenge the thoughts that you are hungry.

Successful applicants of intermittent fasting have their brains always occupied to leave no room for how hungry they are. This would help you overcommit to achieving your desired outcome through fasting.

- **Take zero-calorie drinks**

The main objective of fasting is to allow the body utilize the stored foods for energy. It is, therefore, not advisable to take foods of drinks rich in calories during this period.

Taking beverages like tea and coffee among other drinks that lack calories should be encouraged to avoid dehydration during the fasting process.

- **Never expect miracles**

Intermittent fasting has many roles in our bodies that are not limited to losing extra weight and increasing the insulin sensitivity by our bodies. For the benefits to be experienced, this fasting is just one of the many factors for the desired health benefits. Do not expect to lose about 8% weight simply because you are fasting.

- **Expect discouragements from those around you**

For example, the culture of taking breakfast is so much ingrained to the extent that failing to take it is considered crazy. Most of those around you might try to discourage you against fasting. Having this awareness would be important to help you follow the program to meet your desired health benefits.

- **Regular physical exercise**

Many people see it difficult to go to the gym while fasting not knowing they would be increasing chances for an early achievement of their desired weight. Fasted training can for example result in improved muscle protein synthesis, better metabolic adaptations among other benefits. Have the mentality that fasting would not cause muscle loss during this period.

CHAPTER TWO: History of Intermittent Fasting

Our bodies naturally undergo alternating fasting and feasting. This means that intermittent fasting is part of our livelihood and date back to centuries. I addition to this, even the animals fast as a normal existence course.

For centuries, this fasting has remained effective with the health practitioners, priests, and philosophers using it. For instance, in ancient India and Egypt, voluntary abstaining from food was considered curative, spiritual as well as a preventive intervention against certain conditions.

Since then fasting has remained a religious practice with the Christians, Hindus, Muslims, Taoists, Jainists among other religions.

Christians during the Lent are only allowed to consume the unleavened bread, which was done by Jews long ago during the Pesach or the Passover. During the first two centuries of its existence, fasting was made a voluntary action that entailed receiving the sacraments of the Holy Communion, the ordination of the priests as well as baptism. With time, fasting became an obligation among all Christians. Lenten fast was expanded from its original 40 hours to 4 days with only one meal permitted a day.

Muslims also fast annually during the month of Ramadhan as a form of atonement. They fast from sunrise to sunset during this holy month. Neither food nor fluids are allowed during the fasting period as opposed to many other protocols of fasting. Because of this, they undergo a period of mild dehydration.

The feasting period before sunset and sunrise negates the beneficial effects of this natural therapeutic program because of the increased intake of calories as a result. Considering instructions by the prophet Muhammad, Muslims are also encouraged to fast both on Mondays and on Thursdays of every week.

As a passage of rite, the early man for various important reasons used fasting. Infertility was linked with the anger of the gods and hence fasting was usually done during the autumnal equinoxes to curb the curse. The native Mexicans, as well as the Incas from Peru, also observed fasting to appease their gods.

Historians have come up with publications to illustrate that fasting began a long time ago with our ancestors. Fasting was used to treat the health conditions like the obesity, allergies, high blood pressure and headache among other illnesses.

The ancient Greek historian Herodotus argued that people perceived illness through food. He said that Egyptians were healthy because of their common practice of purification of enemas and vomiting for three days every month.

Plato also realized that fasting was one of the primary treatments. Asclepiad in the 90 BC practiced the use of both the "reorporatsiya" and "metazinkreziya" that entail the use of periodic fasting, bathing, exercising and rubbing.

The ideology of using fasting for health reasons wondered until the middle ages. During this period, people engaged in excessive eating and drinking. This was the reason as to why most of them became severely sick at the age of 40 years. After the miraculous healing of Cornaro, one doctor exclaimed that a strict abstinence from food could help prevent against diseases.

Dr. Chain in the year 1671 to 1743 suggested reforms on the daily diet following recovery from the hell of excessively consuming pork chops and ale.

Today, scientific medicine have become dominant since the drugs were developed. Fasting as a therapeutic intervention fell out of favor in the world. Surprisingly, during this falling out, in Germany, doctors still included the idea of controlled fasting as an integrated medical practice. Dr. Edward Dewey, in the year 1877, was the first person to apply fasting as a mitigation against diseases that involves the loss of appetite and coated tongue. He argued that one should avoid eating once he or she regains his or her appetite and the tongue becomes cleansed for more than 50 days.

However, with the increasing cases of preventable conditions like obesity, several studies have been conducted globally to prove the benefit of fasting in cutting extra weight as well as its psychological effects. Surveillance was done on people with the aim of making a great contribution to the field of science. This led to renewed interest in the reliance in fasting to control the health diseases. Greenfield exclaimed that if people could do a day fast for at least twice a year (one during the spring and one during the autumn), their bodies would mitigate the toxic effects during their daily living.

In support of this natural method, the wide dissemination of therapeutic fasting like the recognized limotherapy further made many health practitioners apply fasting as a medical control practice. Due to this rapid evolution of fasting as a therapeutic intervention in the 21st century, many physicians recommend it for anyone who would wish to have an optimal health regardless of whether he or she is sick or not.

Without forgetting, the hunger strikes experienced among but not limited to the employees against bad leadership.

It is now clear that fasting has remained significant ever since. Fasting has become a means of improving one's health as opposed to the drugs (some with adverse health effects). Most people use fasting as a means of avoiding surgery that might bring complications after that. Let every person develop the belief that fasting among other natural remedies controls the emotions, mental and spiritual aspects of our bodies towards a happy and healthy living.

CHAPTER THREE: Types of Intermittent Fasting

With the research indicating that restricting calories intake is important in increasing the lifespan in humans and other animals, intermittent fasting has been gaining popularity globally for quite some time now. This dieting pattern is not constant in all individual since the health outcomes depend on caloric reduction, hormonal management, decreased hunger as well as the prioritized benefits.

Not taking consideration about how long one stays without eating, intermittent fasting can make one avoid calories intake for between 16 to 36 hours. Further extension of the period over which we fast is what defines this intermittent fasting.

In the mathematical scenario, the vector principle suggests many different routes to the same destination. This is correct when it comes to cutting our bodies off calories for a regulated period. There are different fasting methods that in the end would result in the same health benefits in different people. This is because it is understood that there is no single similarity between two people and that different nutritional approaches would ensure the desired health outcomes are achieved in different individuals.

Each recommended method has its own specific guidelines on what to eat as well as how long our bodies would have to stay without food. It is, therefore, important to choose the best method that you enjoy and believe would work for you.

1. Eat Stop Eat Type of Fasting

This fasting method by Brad Pilon entails avoiding food for up to 24 hours once or twice a week. Just like any other form of fasting, this Eat Stop Eat type of fasting involves eating foods less than what your body is used to. This will, in turn, ensure that the caloric value within the body is cut by a certain percentage.

Most of the fasting techniques require self-discipline in ensuring you achieve the desired outcome. This 24-hour fast, once or twice in every week, however, is flexible since you are the one to decide when to fast as well as when to feast provided it sums to 24 hours of fasting. Opting to fast during your busiest days is the recommended since you do not have time to think about the hunger. The fasting days can as well be adjusted in case of a family event among other planned gatherings to suit your preference.

During this fasting period, only the non-calorific drinks like coffee, tea and water are allowed to protect the body against excessive dehydration. The solid foods are not allowed during this period.

As an important point to note, ensure you normally eat during the feasting time. That is, consume the normal amount of food as if you have not been fasting. Taking more food than normal would render your effort of cutting extra weight useless since you would be experiencing constant undesirable weight gain.

How the 24-hour fasting is done

Just as the name suggests, this type of fasting entails depriving your body of food for a maximum of 24 hours once or twice a week. For example, if you eat today at 8 pm and avoid food until 8 pm the following day, then that is the complete 24-hour fasting technique. Some people might decide to take their meal at 6 am then fast until the following morning. The ultimate outcome would remain the same.

Severe dehydration might occur during this fasting period, and this is the reason why the health practitioners advise us to increase the intake of fluids that are non-calorific to help rehydrate our bodies and as a result avoid the ill effects that might arise from this.

However, just like the other forms of fasting, this 24-hour fasting system remains a challenge to most of the people who would wish to try it for the first time because their bodies are not used to the type of dieting. Some assume that they are entitled to more food during the feasting period because they had fasted. The aforementioned self-control is the virtue that is important in ensuring we all enjoy the benefits of this program.

Research indicate that this is one of the simplest methods we can consider for fasting because once your 24 hours are over, you get back to your normal feeding habit provided you don't overeat.

Advantage of this Eat Stop Eat method of fasting

This type of fasting is one of the most common techniques that people prefer. This is because of some of the advantages that it has recorded over the others.

- **Abstinence from the intake of calories for a longer duration**

Considering most of the fasting forms available, an individual can decide to extend their fasting by just an hour or two. However, this is different with this type of fasting since one has to survive with non-caloric drinks for a longer period of time (24 hours).

This means that with this type of fasting, you lose weight much faster compared to the other forms like the Lean Gain type that requires one only to fast for 14 hours in women and 16 hours in men.

- **This method is easy to adapt**

Fasting is like interfering with the way our bodies operate. It takes our bodies many struggles to work effectively during the fasting period. The 24-hour fasting technique is an easy one since the only rule involved is that one must stay without food for 24 hours.

Unlike most of the fasting types, this method does not limit the amount of food to take during the days you are not fasting. Recent research conducted indicates that this would still ensure a deficit in calories. In addition to this, this Brad's system does not restrict you from taking your favorite foods. This has been a selling factor for this type of fasting.

Compared to some forms that require one to fast for about 36 hours, this Eat Stop Eat strategy is relatively simple, especially for the newbies.

- **This method is flexible**

This point is greatly explained in at the explanatory part of this chapter. This one factor influences how people adopt this fasting technique as a means of losing extra weight among other health benefits.

In this context, flexibility means that you can decide on your favorable time to begin your fast without having to follow the strict orders by the physicians. For example, one decides to begin his or her fasting in the morning or even in the afternoon provided the fasting duration sums to 24 hours.

2. The Alternate-Day Fasting

This type of intermittent fasting requires one to fast on alternating days by either taking fewer calories or none at all to realize its sudden positive effects. This method comes with many versions provided at the end of the day you deny your body food for a specific period. The most common version of this alternate-day fasting involves the 'modified' fasting where one is only allowed to consume only up to about 500 calories counts per fasting day.

Depending on the different people, this form of fasting can involve a person fasting for the whole day or just some hours. Just like illustrated, a full fast is never recommended for those who are trying to fast for the first time.

With this type of fasting, you would be going to be very hungry most of the times a week. This is very unpleasant and might as well have unpleasant effects with time.

This type of intermittent fasting is ideal as a great weight loss instrument and lowering the chances of one getting both the type 2 diabetes and heart conditions.

How to do the alternate-day fasting

Just as the name suggests, you are required to fast for a day then eat whatever you feel like the following day. As a condition in any form of fasting, the only digestible you are required to ingest are the non-caloric beverages like the water and tea among the many others. These are aimed at hydrating our bodies, which constantly dehydrate during the fasting durations.

During the non-fasting periods, you are allowed to eat whatever you desire. This one thing makes this type of fasting a unique and important strategy to ensure your body utilizes the stored energy.

Considering "The Every Other Day," one of the modified ADF strategy, an individual is only required to consume about 25% of his or her general energy requirements. This mostly translates to 500 calories during the fasting days.

Professional nutritionists advise that we include more fruits, vegetables, whole grains, dairy products as well as proteins in our diet during our non-fasting days. This helps our body to be able to have more nutrients to break down during the fasting period the following day.

3. The Warrior Diet as a Fasting Strategy

There are sometimes you feel like eating less during the day and end up eating much at night. This is what The Warrior Diet stands for. Ori Hofmekler was the first to introduce this form of fasting. This form of intermittent fasting was named Warrior diet because of the Warriors' ability to stay up to 20 hours during the day without food and eat a heavy meal during the remaining four hours of the night. With regard to this, the warrior diet entails the undereating during the day that is, fresh juice, raw fruit, few servings of protein as well as vegetable.

This less intake of less food during the day is followed by a heavy meal during the night to help facilitate the body's parasympathetic nervous system in enhancing a calm, relaxed and enhanced digestion.

What you decide to eat and when you are eating it is of great concern when it comes to this type of fasting. It is recommended we begin by consuming vegetables, proteins, and fat in significant quantities. Add carbohydrates in case you still feel hungry. The feasting period must be about four hours.

One unique and important fact about this type of fasting is that it emphasizes on the paleo diet, that is, intake of the unprocessed, whole foods.

According to Hofmekler, the body fats are burnt during the day to produce energy that helps the body produce hormones at night during the heavy feasting.

Benefits of this type of fasting

The fact that this type of fasting allows someone to ingest food in a small amount during the fasting period makes it widely acceptable. This makes it easy to get through unlike the other forms of fasting, which requires one to survive on only the non-caloric drinks or sometimes a dry fast.

During the 20 hours of fasting, the growth hormone is increased and just like any other type of fasting; fewer calories are consumed.

This type of fasting is flexible since, during the four hours of feasting period, the makeup of that food is not important provided adequate protein is consumed. This means that you can as well consume the 'junk' foods and still live a happy and fulfilling life.

In general, having a single meal in a day is economically affordable and hence simple to live by. This, as a result, has led to reduced stress among those who are of less economic status but still desire to drop some weight among the other health benefits of fasting.

Individuals that have tried this type of fasting record increased rates of fat loss as well as the energy levels.

Drawbacks of the warrior diet type of intermittent fasting

Trying to acquire the maximum calories in one meal means that the meal has to be very large that eating would. As a result, lead to discomfort. This fact discourages many people from applying this type of fasting procedure.

Although, it is better since a person is allowed to consume few snacks during the 20 plus fasting hours, following the strict guideline on what needs to be eaten can be hectic to many people.

This fasting form would also cause a headache during planned social gatherings like the family meetings and the wedding ceremonies. It would be tricky for some people to avoid the mouth-watering foods at the expense of just consuming fruits or vegetable.

Other individuals do not have the ability to consume large meals at a time and hence find this type of fasting technique quite discouraging. In addition to this, the following of the strict guideline involved would also not favor their preferences.

4. The 16/8 Method: Fast for 16 hours each day

Martin Berkhan, a fitness expert, popularized this type of fasting.

This type of fasting involves an individual fasting for a maximum of 16 hours with a feasting window of about 8 hours. During the 8 hours, one can have more than one meal depending on their preferences. Women, however, due to their delicate nature, should fast for only a maximum of 14 hours.

Just like any other form of fasting, no consumption of calories is allowed during the fasting period.

Research indicate that most of the users prefer fasting during the night and end up breaking the fast six hours after waking up.

This type of intermittent fasting is ideal and easy for every person provided a specific feeding window is maintained constant. If this is not considered, an undesirable hormone imbalance will result making it difficult to adapt to the new fasting program.

This type of fasting is ideal for the gym-goers. When you work out determines the feeding window. For example, the days you go to the gym requires that you consume more of carbohydrates than fats as compared to increased intake of fats during the resting days. However, the protein intake should remain relatively high every other day depending on gender, body fat, age as well as the desired outcomes of the fast.

Whole, unprocessed foods should consist a larger portion of the meal during the feasting duration. This means that the type of food you eat during the feasting period would determine the general outcome. Eating many junk foods or foods rich in excess calories would not be helpful in achieving your desired weight. Non-caloric drinks like tea and water can be ingested during this fasting window.

Benefits of 16/8 fasting protocol

This type of fasting enhances hormonal management. This is common in all the intermittent fasting programs, but it is far much advanced in this 16/8 fasting procedure. This makes it an ideal program for all.

Within the 8-hour feasting period, you can eat whatever you wish. Taking three meals during the feeding period makes it easy for those who try this type of fasting. For a comfortable and successful fasting, this is one of the best fasting methodologies.

During the fasting periods, the feeling of hunger is a common experience. This is not the case when it comes to this type of intermittent fasting. Recent studies indicate that the 16/8 fasting form has a hunger management advantage. The infrequent meals involved make you feel fuller for a longer period.

Drawbacks of the 16/8 fasting procedure

Unlike the other forms of fasting, this type of fasting is effective when one does workouts in a fasted state. This makes it hectic for those individuals that hate engaging in physical exercises.

The difficulty in following the simple nutrition plans when it comes to this type of fasting forces many people to shift the feasting duration to inconvenient intervals. This also applies to what we eat in relation to the type of activities you engage in during this time.

5. Fat Loss Forever Intermittent Fasting Method

This fasting method is branded a 'hybrid' since it was developed following the combination of all the three most common types of fasting: the Warrior Diet, Eat Stop Eat, and the Lean Gains methods. This was the work of Dan Go and Romaniello to utilize the strengths of every individual fasting methods while ruling out their weaknesses. According to the plan by your professional instructor, a specific intermittent fasting technique is followed on certain days. Until you meet your desired outcomes.

This method is ideal for those who desire to lose more weight within a limited period. This is possible when you engage in this type of fasting for a period of 12 weeks.

It is advisable that you engage in longer fasts on the days that you are very busy since you have no space to think about how hungry you are.

Benefits of Fat Loss Forever IF Method

Since it involves a combination of all the three outstanding fasting methods, this cocktail type of fasting ensures that you achieve your goals within limited time. For the controlled 12-week program, significant outcomes are observed. This is the reason why this type is important for those individuals that are never patient.

Advanced hormonal management. Combining the three types of fasting would increase the concentration of growth hormone within the body and hence the related benefits.

Drawbacks of Fat Loss Forever IF Method

This become a more complicated system to follow for those individuals who are not able to follow the strict guidelines of the individual fasting methods. This is because, during the stipulated duration of the fasting program, each individual fasting method is considered on specific days.

Some people use this type of fasting as an excuse to eat the processed, unwholesome meals. This makes many people not to enjoy the benefits of this Fat Loss Forever IF Method.

In conclusion

With the many types of intermittent fasting, not limited to the once mentioned above, it is important to consult a health professional to help you choose the best strategy that fits you. This would be the first step once you realize that this strategy would simplify your nutrition. This is because people have varying personalities and chemical composition hence different techniques would work for each one of them.

Personal experimentation can also be helpful when it comes to determining the ideal method that fits you. Consider trying each method at different times to ensure you achieve your desired outcome.

It is good to choose the method that makes you comfortable since there is no form of fasting that would produce positive results when you feel miserable and stressed out.

CHAPTER FOUR: Benefits of Intermittent Fasting

This belief that meal skipping leaves our bodies in a starvation mode has proved to be a great challenge in the campaign about fasting as a health remedy for various conditions. This is possible because of the cut calories which allows our body to utilize the stored energy for the normal cell functioning. The benefits of the fasting supplements like the vegetables, nuts, fruits and fish among others make this strategy an important weapon against diseases.

The stigmatization that comes along with this meal skipping tendency has made the health practitioners to avoid as much as possible giving this strategy as an intervention against the health problems. This, however, does not undermine the incredible benefits that come along with this practice. This is because of the mounting evidence that other key aspects of diet (how and when often people eat) play an important role in a healthy lifestyle.

A. Fasting helps in losing extra weight

There are many ways to lose weight. According to different studies, intermittent fasting proves to be one of the ideal ways in losing some extra body mass. This is because the body is allowed to burn the fat cells to produce the energy used within the body. This would not be the case during the normal dieting since the ingested calories would be the ones broken down instead.

To further support the importance of skipped meals on weight loss, this intermittent fasting is known to facilitate the hormone functioning that enhances the loss of weight. That is, reduced calories intake would result in low insulin levels, increased noradrenaline as well as a higher growth hormone levels. This hormone optimization increases the rate at which our bodies act on the body fat to be the ultimate energy source. Fortunately, we end up losing the extra mass thereby achieving our desired weight reading.

Introducing your body to the actual intermittent fasting elevates the body metabolic rate by about 14% to facilitate the fast burning of the body fat. It is clear that this would result in a loss of some pounds of mass.

With the above explanation, it is clear that intermittent fasting is helpful when in need of losing some mass since calories intake is limited. This is also possible due to our boosted metabolic rate.

Research conducted in 2014 indicates that about 8% of weight is lost between 3-24 weeks of intermittent fasting. This important factor has triggered many individuals to try this remedy for a successful venture. This was supported by the loss of about 4-7% loss of the waist circumference indicating that the belly fat responsible for frequent abdominal pain among those with heavy bodies is burnt.

As a caution, this method would not result in loss of weight if you opt to compensate the fasting period by eating much during the non-fasting periods.

B. Intermittent fasting promotes longevity

Though it is difficult to believe, the less you eat, the longer you might live. This is supported by most studies that show a higher life expectancy among those who have the culture of skipping meals than those who enjoy all the meals.

This type of fasting boosts our immunity and the restorative properties of the body. This ensures that we live a longer and enjoyable life with no fear of dying anytime soon.

This was supported by research done on the c. Elegans worm that have some genes that we too have. The research indicated an increased longevity if subjected to similar intermittent fasting conditions.

It is clear that fasting reduces the insulin concentration within the body of an individual. Brain insulin signaling reduction has been seen to further increase the longevity by literally knocking the brain insulin receptor out or by calorie restricting. This is also recognized in rats.

A healthy lifestyle is connected to increased longevity. This means that relying on intermittent fasting has a means of enhancing our health by burning the belly fat, for example, would. As a result, translate to increased longevity.

Aging is associated with a slow rate of metabolism. This means that the younger you look, the higher the metabolism rate. Cutting the introduction of calories within the body would facilitate an increased metabolic process since it takes less time for the little food ingested to be digested. This slows down the aging rate of an individual.

For a long and happy life, it is important to consider this special intervention that has a proven track record from recent studies.

C. Intermittent fasting with heart health

Researchers indicate that heart problem is one of the killer diseases in the world today. In connection to this, the elites argue that the various risk factors are connected to either a decreased or increased chances of heart disease. Such health markers include the blood pressure, the blood triglycerides, the LDL cholesterol and the inflammatory markers among other factors.

However, this intermittent fasting has been proven to harmonize these risk factors for a healthy heart. This is possible because those who fast have control over the amount of calorie they take into their bodies and this then translates to better and healthy heart due to the favorable eating choices.

The rate at which our bodies metabolize the cholesterol within the body determines the heart health. Regular intermittent fasting increases the body metabolic rate. This ensures that the bad cholesterol is broken down as fast as possible to minimize the risks of heart diseases by reducing the risks of gaining extra weight and diabetes.

If you need to begin a fast with the intention of maintaining a healthy heart, consult your personal physician on the types of foods or drinks to use as a supplement during your fasting periods. Maintaining a heart-healthy diet and regular physical exercises further improves the general health.

Lowering the levels of fat within the body because of intermittent fasting lessens the kidney workload hence a lower blood pressure. This lowered blood pressure as well as the increased production of the growth hormone enhances an effective cardiac function.

D. The role of intermittent fasting in the war against cancer

Cancer is a chronic disease that is characterized by the abnormal cell growths. Intermittent fasting, therefore, has been seen as an important arsenal to help in the killing of cancer cells.

During this period, the normal cells 'hibernates' while the cancerous cells continue multiplying trying to find alternative survival means but without any success.

As a common measure against cancer, the normal cells were found to have the ability to withstand the chemotherapy. This therapy is best done when the body is in a starvation mode to easily differentiate the healthy cells from the cancerous ones.

Regardless of its remedy against cancer, intermittent fasting is not a strategy that every cancer patients can rely on. For example, those patients who have lost about 10% of their total body weight or have chronic conditions such as diabetes should not subject themselves to fasting. This can be so disastrous to the health of the individual.

It is, therefore, important to consult your physician to enable you to understand the stage of your condition before turning to fasting as the ultimate intervention against cancer.

E. Fasting improves the immune system

Considering all the health benefits that come along with fasting, it is correct to argue that it boosts our bodies in the fight against diseases. These health effects result when the free radicles are reduced, the cancerous cells starved and the inflammatory condition regulated. These effects only occur when our bodies are in the state of fast.

As an illustration, when an animal is sick it does not feed. This action minimizes the pressure on the internal body system in the war against diseases.

During fasting, a regenerative switch gives an 'OK' for the stem cells to create new white cells. The body, as a result, gets rid of the damaged cells during this period. This entire procedure facilitates the creation of literally a new immune system.

Records indicate that individuals who fast for about four days in every six months experience limited cases of infections.

During this starvation period, the body tries to save energy by recycling the unused or damaged white cells.

F. Health benefits of intermittent fasting for the brain

Since our body organs are interconnected, whatever benefits the body would as well benefit the brain. This, therefore, means that the different types of fasting are beneficial when it comes to brain health.

When subjecting yourself to any form of intermittent fasting, the metabolism rates aimed at reducing the oxidative stress, reducing the blood sugar levels, insulin resistance as well as reduced inflammation. These physiological processes are helpful when it comes to a healthy brain in humans and animals in general.

This fasting increases the levels of the brain-derived neurotrophic factor hormones. The level of this hormone lowers during depression along with other various brain complications. This increase in the level of these hormones indicates that the brain is in its favorable state.

This skipping of meals facilitates the growth of nerve cells within the brain to enhance the brain functioning.

G. Spiritual importance of intermittent fasting

The one thing that most people know is that fasting is a means of losing extra mass to achieve the desired body weight. This is not the case when it comes to religion. Nearly every religion values the role of fasting in bringing them close to their Supreme Being.

In a religious setup, fasting is not necessarily meant for health benefits but as a means of showing faith in your beliefs. Fasting entails saying an 'NO' to the natural appetite to be close to God the Almighty. For example, Muslims fast during the month of Ramadhan as a directive by Prophet Mohamed to enhance their purifications. Christians, Hindus, Puritans among all the other spiritual religions do fast for reasons such as famine or even drought.

The spiritual fasting also helps in discovering the self-awareness of an individual. This is an early and quick track to discover where your addiction and truth lie.

The Side Effects of Intermittent Fasting

Intermittent fasting record both the positive and negative impacts. This depends on the individual hormonal stability as well as the type of fasting method employed.

Any intervention that is introduced comes with its own guiding principles. Acting against these principles would mean you experience the undesirable outcome. This is the same when it comes to all methods of fasting.

I. Obsession with the feeding and fasting window

Since intermittent fasting entails alternating periods of fasting and feasting, some individuals tend to get obsessed with when the feasting time would come. They end up thinking about food as a result.

To make this worse, some dieters fail to follow the IF standard guidelines and end up extending their fast period to observe an immediate outcome. In the end, unhealthy weight loss results that is later regained.

The reason why most obsessed dieters regain their weight is that they eventually go back to their old eating habits.

II. The feeling of starvation

Food cravings and hunger are some of the usual challenges when someone is trying to cut some mass off for healthy living. Hunger pangs have been observed in some individuals who eat six meals during the non-fasting period.

The feeling of hunger is an early sign when you begin your fasting journey to enjoy the benefits that follow. Your body adapts to the state with a time of regular controlled fasting.

III. Caffeine addiction

Intermittent fasting allows the consumption of non-caloric beverages to enable the dieters to remain energized and rehydrated. Such drinks include coffee, water, and tea. Both the coffee and tea contain caffeine that is addictive to users. Dieters end up over-relying on the coffee and tea.

Addiction to these drinks is associated with stress, anxiety and poor sleeping habit, which as a result leads to the undesirable regaining of weight.

IV. Reduces athletic performance

Though it is advisable to engage in lighter exercise during the fasting period to realize faster weight loss, intense workouts have been found to cause injury to the dieter. In addition to this, exercising during the fasting period causes extra fatigue than usual.

V. Headaches

Due to the stress that we expose our body to during this fasting period, headaches are common experiences. This is the reason why non-caloric drinks are allowed during the fasting region. For example, drinking water was seen to relieve the headaches in some cases.

VI.   Imbalanced hormone in women

Missed periods, early-onset menopause and metabolic disturbances are some of the negative effects that intermittent fasting have on women. This is because women hormones are very sensitive to energy intake. Long fasting hours would, therefore, interfere with the hormones. To curb this, professionals advice that women try the modified form of intermittent fasting (crescendo).

The side effects above are not for a specific type of intermittent fasting. It is, therefore, vital to consult your physicians to help you select the best fasting strategy to lose the extra weight.

CHAPTER FIVE: Women and Intermittent Fasting

With the increased campaign on the role of intermittent fasting as a means of cutting off extra weight among the several other health benefits, it was discovered that women were extremely sensitive to starvation and hence responded differently to this skipping of meals. That is, fasting might result to a hormonal imbalance and hence fertility problems in women if not done correctly. This is the body's way of protecting the fetus (even when we are not expectant). This affects women as young as in their mid-20s.

Scientific studies indicate that prolonged calories deficit, as well as reduced fat mass, might lead to different forms of menstrual dysfunction (amenorrhea) as well as decreased estradiol, insulin and leptin levels among women.

Fasting and the female hormones

In both women and men, hypothalamic-pituitary-gonadal axis acts systematically. The hypothalamus first releases the gonadotropin hormone that in turn triggers the pituitary gland to produce both the follicular stimulating hormone and the luteinizing hormone. Both the LH and the FSH act as gonads (testes in men or ovaries in women). In women, for example, these gonads facilitate the production of both the estrogen and progesterone in women to help in ovulation.

Women, unlike men, experience very specific and regular hormonal cycles. This, therefore, means that the gonadotropin hormones have to be timed to avoid getting the physiological function out of balance. The GnRH are sensitive to environmental determinants including the simple skipping of meals. This, therefore, calls for a gentle and controlled implementation of the intermittent fasting strategy.

The kisspeptin, a protein that is made in the hypothalamus, is responsible for the production of the gonadotropin hormones in both women and men for proper reproductive functions. Because of the more kisspeptin in women than in males, hence a greater sensitivity to insulin, ghrelin and leptin-the hormones that react to satiety and hunger.

The normal signs of a hormonal imbalance when in a starvation mode

1) The feeling of fatigue.

This feeling normally occurs because of respiration in a limited supply of oxygen. Engaging in uncontrolled fasting might affect the normal functioning of the hormones responsible for the breaking down of the accumulated lactic acid within the body tissues.

2) The feeling of depression

This feeling of hopelessness results when you engage in different forms of fasting with no significant outcome. The failure of your body to benefit from fasting is due to the altered normal hormonal balancing.

Among the other signs of an altered hormonal functioning are a headache, irregular periods and bloating.

To curb this, scientists argue that fasting on nonconsecutive days might be useful in maintaining the hormones in check among the women. This is known as the Crescendo type of fasting since you try the different fasting methods until you identify the suitable one that matches your body system.

The crescendo intermittent fasting for women

Jumping into intermittent fasting for the women can be very hard due to their characteristic hormone fluctuating levels. It is, therefore, important for the newbies to consider a modified intermittent type of fasting (crescendo).

This type of fasting requires that a woman fasts on nonconsecutive days. The hormones do not go frenzy when one applies this type of meal skipping.

The modified fasting technique is a more gentle approach in ensuring the women adapt to fasting. Done right, this can be a great remedy in ensuring you lose some extra mass without altering the hormonal balance as a result.

Though Crescendo type of fasting is not necessary for all women, it can be successful when some of the following rules are taken into consideration.

> ➢ **Skip meals for about 2-3 nonconsecutive days.**

Professionals advise that during the fasting days, the woman engages herself for about sixteen hours. It is also important to engage in physical exercise during the fasting period. The exercise should be less intense.

> ➤ **Drink non-caloric beverages during the fasting period**

During this fasting period, the amount of calories taken is cut to allow the body utilize the stored fats for energy. Non-caloric drinks such as water, tea, and coffee among others should be consumed to rehydrate the body after dehydration during this fasting period.

> ➤ **Eat normally when under a high-cardio day**

When engaging in heavy training, one can be tempted to compensate the lost energy by eating more food than he or she eats on the normal days. This helps the body adapt to the starvation state with time.

> ➤ **Add an additional fasting day**

After about two weeks of fasting, when you feel comfortable, it is good to extend your weekly fasting by a day to help the body get used to the starvation mode as quick as possible. This is optional depending on the desires of the woman who needs to experiment this special fasting strategy.

> ➤ **Taking about 8 grams of BCAAs during your fasting period**

The BCAAs amino acid supplement contains fewer calories that remain vital in providing the energy for the muscle development. This is also helpful in edging off the feeling of hunger or fatigue during this period. Though it is also optional, supplementing your body with these amino acids protects the muscles from being burnt down during this fasting period.

> **When to stop fasting**

In case you notice any sign of hormonal imbalance, for example, irregular menstrual cycles or sometimes the eating disorders, stop the fasting immediately. This could mean that the common intermittent fasting is not recommended for you. This is, however, never the case if the procedure is done gently and professionally.

This Crescendo style of fasting is recommended for the women who react adversely to the other forms of fasting. For our women to remain healthy during their fasting periods, it is important to engage in this modified intermittent fasting technique.

CHAPTER SIX: Intermittent Fasting and Caloric Restriction

With the desire to live a longer and happy life, many individuals have turned to reducing the amount of food let into their bodies. This is done professionally to avoid malnutrition. This is what is termed as the caloric restriction. In detail, this caloric restriction entails reducing the total calories count by about 30% to 40% the standard daily requirement. This calories restriction is not fun for either humans or other animals.

Intermittent fasting, on the other hand, involves staying for extra durations without having any food. This can be considered the latest form of caloric restriction strategies since an individual willingly decides to avoid eating for some specific period to experience some of its health benefits. This means that one who subjects himself or herself to intermittent fasting would ultimately lengthen his or her life. There are many different forms of intermittent fasting to choose from.

Similarities between Intermittent Fasting and Calories Restrictions

Just like mentioned above, Intermittent fasting is one of the most recent forms of calories restrictions, if not the most recent. This means that both the CR and IF have some similar principles that define them.

a) Both of them undergo the fasting and feasting periods

Just like the intermittent fasting, caloric restriction involves feeding at the specific period as well as starving for some period. For example, after long hours of hunger, those under caloric restriction tend to eat much food. Feeding once in a day when under the CR, is equivalent to having fasted for about 24 hours each day.

b) They are both aimed at enhancing a longer life

Studies indicate that the fat tissues have an indirect connection with a longer life. The CR's principle desire to increase longevity forces it to, therefore, act on the adipose tissues in order to reduce the fat content.

This is similar to intermittent fasting, which allows the body to burn the stored fats as the alternative source of energy. This reduced fat mass would result in a life-extending effect among those under the program.

c) The importance of physical exercise

The common mouse, the most preferred specimen for scientific studies, does not die of similar diseases as humans. This brings a lot of concern on further studies to exhaust all the factors linked with mortality.

Physicians, as a result, observed that engaging in regular exercises when under restricted calories intake has a synergistic effect on both the inflammation and insulin. Physical exercise, however, would be important in ensuring a longer and healthy life.

d) Both of them involve the feeling of hunger

Caloric restriction just like intermittent fasting alternates the feasting and fasting periods. During the period when you are not eating, the feeling of hunger dominates your body system. What is entailed during this starving period is now what differentiate between the CR from the IF. For instance, in intermittent fasting, drinking of non-caloric beverages is allowed during the fasting period whereas, in other caloric restriction strategies, one is expected to avoid any meal or drinks until the feasting time comes.

e) Both the IF and the CR protect the body against diseases

Increased accumulation of fat within the body tissues is linked to lifestyle conditions such as obesity. These diseases lower the quality of life. This might also lead to mortality, which is against the main principles of both the intermittent type of fasting and calories restrictions. The aim of the two programs is to reduce the amount of fat within the body, therefore, protecting the body against ailments.

Reasons Why Intermittent Fasting Is More Important Than the Calories Restriction Program

Despite the fact that both the strategies are aimed at ensuring life-extension, there must be some specific components that make the two strategies different. The two strategies work differently to ensure they achieve their individual goals of a long and healthy life. For example, caloric reduction entails both the decreased metabolism and the increased appetite while the intermittent fasting, however, involves both the increased metabolism and decreased appetite.

Comparing the two programs, researchers indicate that intermittent fasting is more reliable, in your quest to lengthen life, than the caloric restriction due to several factors.

✓ Intermittent fasting lacks many side effects

Although caloric restriction has the benefit of lengthening the life, it depletes the growth, thyroid and insulin hormones. This CR also manifests as poor cardiac health as well as reducing fertility and libido.

However, intermittent fasting when controlled results in achievement of your desired weight among other health benefits. Your safety is only guaranteed when you choose the best intermittent fasting methods available. It is, therefore, important to visit your physician to guide you through the whole program successfully.

✓ Provides similar metabolic benefits to caloric restriction

Like explained earlier, both the intermittent fasting and caloric restriction programs aim at lengthening life. In geography, the vector principle states that different routes might lead to the same destination. The counselors, however, advise that you choose the best between the two strategies: CR and IF in your quest to achieve a life-extension.

Intermittent fasting, which lacks many negative effects is the best of the two to achieve your desire. Do not end up solving a problem while causing a new one. Consider the IF over the CR for healthy living.

✓ Intermittent fasting provides an additional metabolic boosting

Intermittent fasting, in addition to losing weight, protects the body against metabolic damages. This will ensure that all the nutrients are utilized to produce energy for the basic metabolism.

✓ Intermittent fasting is easily manageable than caloric restriction

The ultimate goals of both the IF and CR are to lengthen life. Intermittent fasting, however, has easy-to-follow guidelines in ensuring you meet your set target. For example, it is advisable to take non-caloric drinks such as water and tea to rehydrate your body during the fasting period.

In general

Intermittent fasting is a form of caloric restriction that is aimed at ensuring life-extension. The two programs use different principles to attain the same results. This, therefore, means that there is no difference between the two programs.

CHAPTER SEVEN: FAQS about Intermittent Fasting

Intermittent fasting has gained popularity globally due to the evidence-based health benefits that come along with it. To understand better what it entails, many questions have been asked by the lovers of this fasting program. This chapter tries to identify some of the frequently asked questions and provide the relevant responses.

1. What does this intermittent fasting entail?

This program gives the body time to utilize the extra energy it stored. The main principle behind this eating pattern is to allow the body to undergo through alternating fasting and feasting cycles to cut the intake of calories as a result.

2. What is the difference between intermittent fasting and caloric restriction?

The CR and the IF tend to share some principles making it difficult for people to distinguish them. Both focuses on the need to lower the intake of calories to enhance a longer and healthy life.

Intermittent fasting is a form of caloric restriction that is controlled.

3. How do I get started?

Several methods of intermittent fasting have been proven to work effectively as weight-loss tools. Some of the fasting methods include but not limited to the following:

- ❖ The Warrior Diet - involving taking a single meal daily
- ❖ Lean Gains - this involves fasting for about 16 hours then break your meals between the feasting duration of 8 hours.
- ❖ Eat Stop Eat - this is a 24-hour fasting either once or twice in every week.
- ❖ An alternate-day fasting – this involves engaging in fasting on alternating days.
- ❖ The Fast-5 Method – this type entails an individual taking 5 hours between their meals.

To get started. Therefore, it is important to consult professionals and choose the best method that benefits you since each method works well in different people.

4. Who can benefit from intermittent fasting?

With the associated benefits that come along with this program, different types of individuals can adapt to the intermittent program. You should be able to enjoy the outcome provided your professional dietician makes you choose the method that fits you.

5. Am I allowed to eat what I want during the feasting period?

After a long duration of fasting, it is good to eat normal as if you were not fasting. Avoid trying to compensate the fast by eating more than you are used to. This normally depends on an individual's lifestyle regarding your daily energy expenditure and food preference and quality. Many individuals need a larger amount of calories to sustain them during the 16-hour fast than for example if you are fasting less than 16 hours. That also depends on your purpose of intermittent fasting such as rapid body weight loss or if you are practicing fasting for spiritually reasons.

6. Can I drink water during my fasting period?

The main aim of this type of fasting is to reduce or cut down the intake of calories to force the body to break down its energy reservoir preferably excess body fat to be the ultimate energy source. During this time, the body can become extremely dehydrated.

Therefore, drinking water among other non-caloric beverages such as tea and coffee are allowed to help in the body's rehydration. However, you need to be careful with coffee and other drinks that contain caffeine since they are diuretics meaning they make you urinate more frequently causing more loss of body fluid thus making you thirsty.

7. Is intermittent fasting advisable for the weightlifters?

Having in mind that fasting breaks down the excess fat within the body to achieve a leaner body and healthier lifestyle, engaging in regular physical exercises such as strength training would further facilitate the burning of fat stored within the body system and maintain or even possible gain muscle tissue.

8. Is it good to have a cheat day?

Some fasting methods such as the 8-hour Diet for seven days is difficult to follow hence up to four cheats in a week is acceptable. These cheat days can work for you, but you should be careful to avoid these cheats since they can lessen the effect of intermittent fast benefits.

9. Can fasting lead to muscle loss?

This should not worry you much since the different methods of intermittent facilitate the breaking down of fats and not the muscles. This would only work when you fully have control of the fasting program. To prevent or minimize muscle loss you should be eating high-quality foods (fats, protein, and carbohydrates) preferably animal based food if you are not a vegan. That way when you start your fasting cycle your body and in particular your muscles are nourished with a complete profile of amino acids from animal based protein. The other components are adding strength workout during the intermittent fasting and doing the strength workout at the end of the IF, so when you break up the fast, you can replenish your muscle tissues with glycogen, protein, and fats.

10. What happens when you fast for 3 days in a raw?

Alternate-day fasting discourages against fasting for consecutive days. However, depending on your lifestyle and preference, there are no ill effects on skipping meals for three or more successive days.

11. Can I take snacks during my fasting period?

The feelings of thirst and hunger develop in the hypothalamus. Either of the feelings can be so tempting during the fasting period. In the case of this, just like mentioned earlier, consider filling your belly with non-caloric beverages such as limewater, hot tea or even coffee.

12. Is intermittent fasting a form of starvation?

Starvation means an extreme malnutrition due to a deficiency in caloric intake within the body. This can be so disastrous to the general health of an individual. In intermittent fasting, however, calories are stored within the body in the form of fat to produce sufficient energy to the body when broken down.

13. Who is not advisable to practice intermittent fasting?

Although IF has been practiced by humans for millennia and very possible, it is part of our human evolution since our ancestor's hunters, and gatherers did not have a stable and guaranteed amount of foods during the different seasons. However, it is advisable not to practice fasting if you are:

-Pregnant since you need to nourish yourself and the baby thus it is not a good time to do that.

-Breastfeeding is very taxing on the mom's body beside the baby needs all the possible nourishment that comes from mom.

-Individuals who have a high amount of stress due to many reasons such as work project completion and other unfortunate situations that are causing a high amount of stress. Your body most likely needs as much help from nutrition at this time. Therefore, it is not advisable to fast.

-Individuals with certain health disorders such as diabetes and other health concerns should consult with their qualified health practitioners and see if intermittent fasting be practiced or not.

CHAPTER EIGHT: Conclusion

Because of the health effects that come along with the stored fat within the body tissue, researchers worked hard to come up with strategies to burn them as the source of fuel within the body. Limiting the calories intake into the body meant that the body had to work on the stored fats to facilitate the basic metabolism. This is a caloric restriction. As a form of caloric restriction, intermittent fasting (an eating pattern that alternated the fasting period and the feasting period) has recently become common in the fight against lifestyle conditions like obesity.

Fasting is a historic process since our ancestors fasted because they either lacked food or for religious reasons. Without knowing, our bodies undergo fasting when we are asleep. In addition to this, the moment we are not eating, we are fasting. This, therefore, means that fasting is a natural process vital for our daily survival.

There are many forms of intermittent fasting that work well with different people: Eat Stop Eat, Alternate-Day Fasting, The Warrior Diet, The 16/8 Methods and Fat Loss Forever. Each intermittent fasting technique works well with different individuals and hence the need to consult professionals before selecting the fasting methodology that would be of help to your health.

Women, for example, experiences frequent hormonal imbalance and hence a modified type of intermittent fasting (crescendo fasting) is the most preferred.

Supplementation like the taking of non-caloric beverages during the fasting period is necessary to rehydrate the body.

A number of benefits come with the correct identification of the most favorable form of fasting. Such include both the spiritual and health benefits. The main aim of fasting is to lose the extra weight hence ensuring a long and healthy living. In addition to this, strong immunity is connected to a successful fasting program.

If not done correctly, fasting can have many adverse effects such as heartburns, headaches, frequent diarrhea and infertility among the many others. Engaging in any fasting program, therefore, requires knowledge of the best method of meal skipping as well as how to do it right for the realization of positive outcomes.

With the global spreading of intermittent fasting as a tool of losing some extra weight, there are many concerns that have arisen from the lovers. This book provides responses to some of the most common questions that are asked for a better understanding of this form of caloric restriction.

Therefore, to record positive results out of the fasting program, consult professionals and choose the best strategy that ensures maximum output. Stay healthy by cutting down the intake of calories.

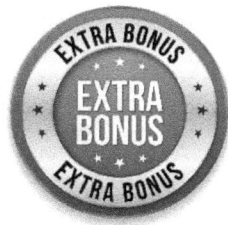

Chapter

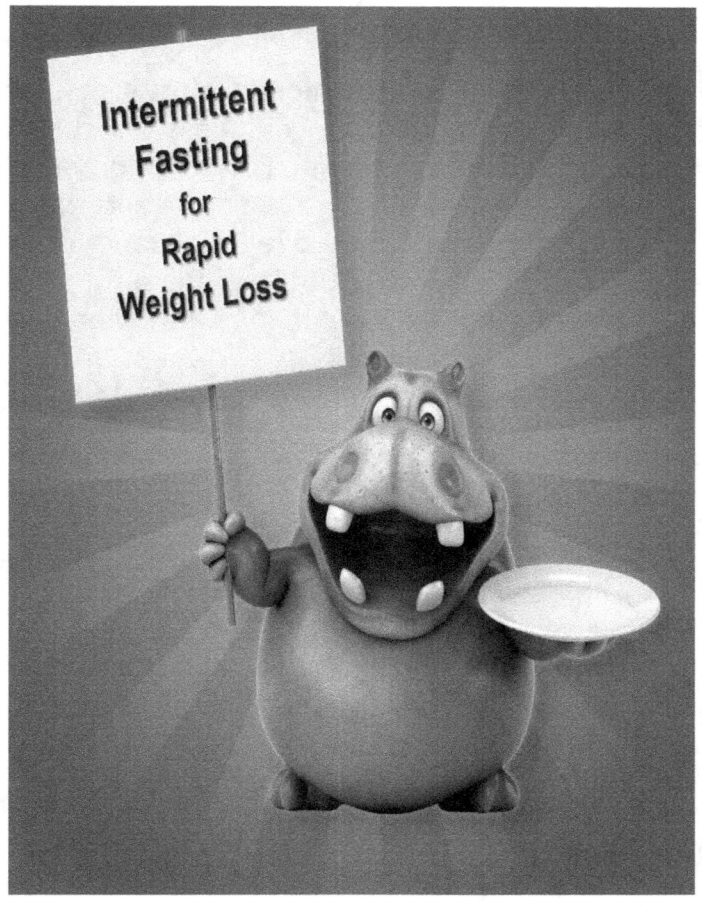

Specific Weight Loss Program Utilizing Intermittent Fasting

As I shared with you in this book, there are different benefits from practicing intermittent fasting however in this chapter I am going to share with you how to optimize your chance to lose weight and specifically body fat while you are practicing IF.

Losing weight can happen almost effortlessly during intermittent fasting practice nevertheless that does not happen with everyone who practices IF unfortunately for various reasons. Although I can't guarantee a hundred percent that you will lose weight and have the same results that I had. But I will share with you effective strategies that you can follow and hopefully you will see noticeable results in few weeks and convert you to an IF believer sooner than later.

Strategy One: Intermittent Fasting with Ketogenic or Low carb/high-fat meals

Some individuals eat meals that are high in carbohydrates and low in fat and possibly low in protein as well. Switching to Keto diet or even low-carb meals might be more effective in making your body to use body fat (ketones) as energy, and gradually but surely you will start to shed off the excess body fat and maintain your muscle tissue.

If you are interested in learning more about ketogenic or low-carb diets you can get my book, All About Ketogenic Diet and will teach you about this topic and how to go about it.

Following Ketogenic diet is stricter than a low-carb diet since you want to force your body to use ketones. When you consume keto diet, your liver will convert fat into ketone bodies and fatty acids.

And likely you will improve the body cells to become less insulin resistance. One possible reason is that you are not bombarding your body with so many carbohydrates (particularly the highly processed ones), leading to, too much insulin secretion, and eventually your cells become resistant to insulin except fat cells.

Another reason for the Ketogenic diet is that can be more satiating due to the high content of fat and moderate amount of proteins which can lead to being satisfied and eating less amount of food and calories. Combine that with intermittent fasting, and you will have a very effective strategy for rapid weight loss.

Examples of Ketogenic and low-carb foods with Pictures

The below images will give you an idea what types of foods to eat and to integrate with your intermittent fasting in order to achieve rapid weight loss outcome.

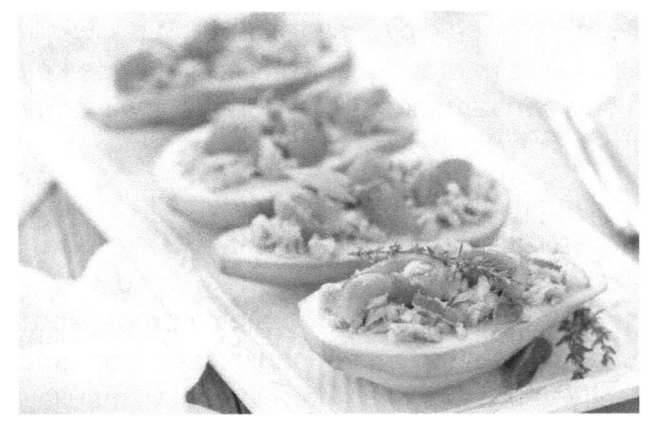

Figure 1 Avocado tuna and tomato salad

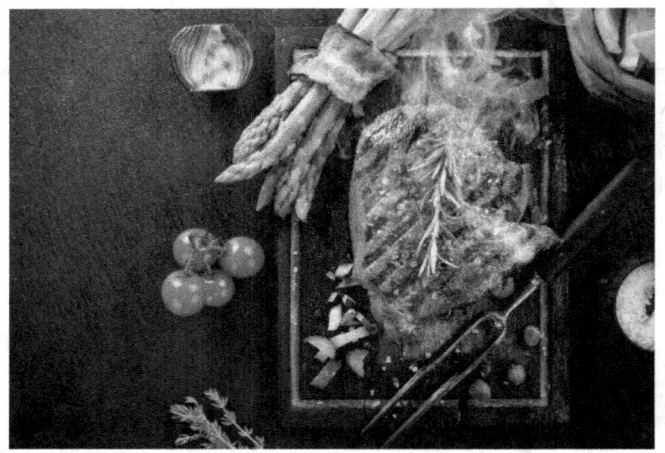

Figure 2 Beef steak with low Starchy Vegetables

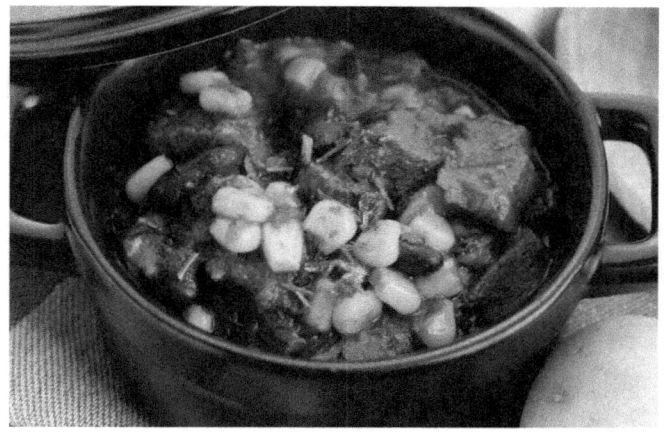

Figure 3 Beef Stew with Vegetables or Beans

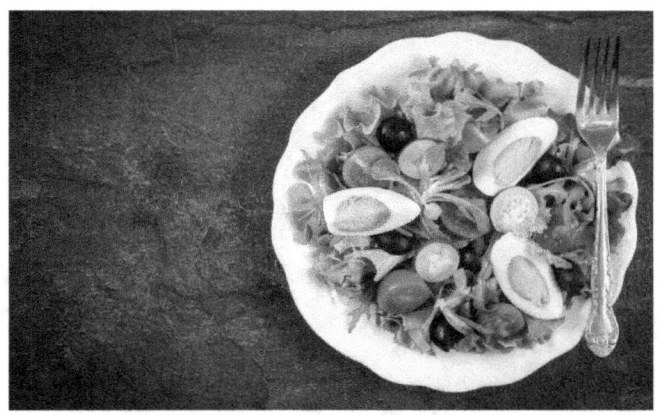

Figure 4 Boiled eggs salad

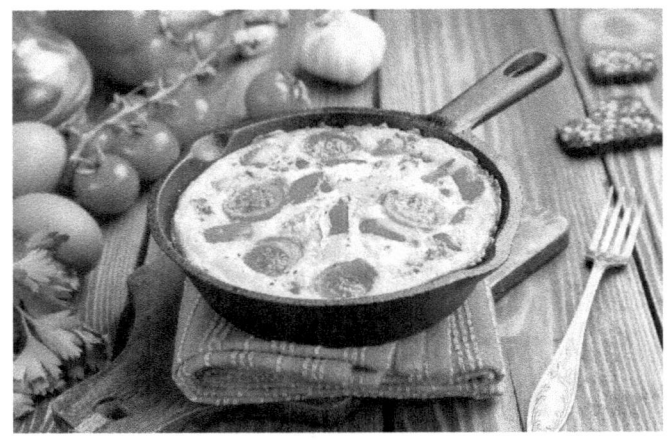

Figure 5 Cheese Bacon Tomato Frittata Keto diet

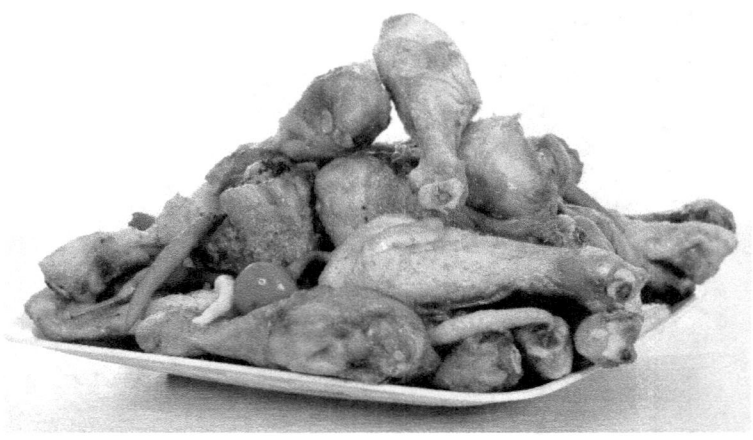

Figure 6 Chicken Drumsticks with sour cream dip

Strategy Two: Resistance Training with Intermittent Fasting

For this strategy, you include a type of resistance training to see rapid weight loss results during intermittent fasting. However, timing is critical here where you want to perform your resistance training at the end of your fasting period.

So if you are fasting for 16 hours, then I would recommend you exercise the last hour or two-hour period.

Fasting = 16 hours	Exercising During the 15th or 16th hour

I performed my resistance training like that for few reasons:

1-I am more likely to use ketones (body fat) since I have been fasting for many hours and I am almost at the end of my fasting cycle.

2-Once I am done with my resistance training, I am soon going to feast or break my fast and replenish my muscles with desperately needed nutrients. Therefore, I am preserving my muscle tissue or even gaining some more, and I have used body fat as energy to workout.

3-It is no fun to perform resistance training, and after you have completed your workout, you still have many hours to wait before completing your intermittent fasting, trust me on that.

Aerobics vs. Resistance Training vs. HIIT During IF

As you have noticed, I mentioned performing resistance training and not aerobics or cardio since it did not yield good results for my clients and me and in particular the female clients. Your resistance workout can be performed at the gym if you like but it can also be done at home with no issues what so ever,

You can also perform High-Intensity Interval Training which is known as HIIT (pronounced as "hit.") and possibly can see even better results than resistance training, but in my experience, that was not necessary, and for many individuals, the HIIT type of training can be very challenging during intermittent fasting.

The idea of including resistance training is to stimulate muscle growth and burn fat using ketone bodies during the fasting period. And the sweet thing here is you will replenish your muscles with some glycogen, fatty acids, and amino acids soon enough since your about a few minutes away from breaking your intermittent fasting.

How to Effectively Perform Resistance Training from Home

Many people think that they have to get a gym membership and use the gym exercise machines to have an effective workout, that's not true for the average person and even beyond the average person. However, this book and this bonus are focused on IF and how to lose bodyweight fast so I will provide you with some exercise names and you can search for them on youtube or the internet. But trust me, these bodyweight exercises can be very demanding, and at the same time, you can adjust them to suit your fitness level.

- All types of pushups (There are at least five varieties I can think of)
- Bodyweight squats
- Lunges
- Pullups
- The good old jumping jack exercise
- The Bear crawl
- Climbing or hiking an uphill for outdoors
- Climbing the stairs in your house
- Step-up exercise
- The walkout exercise
- Sprinting for outdoors training
- Using Resistance bands or tubes at home for pull-down or pull-in
- Resistance tubes for Core exercises

Here you go, try one of the strategies and see which one will work more effectively for you regarding rapid body weight loss during your intermittent fasting and stay with it for as long as you wish. I do however advise that you take a break from doing both at the same time, the IF and Resistance Training or HIIT to give yourself a mental and physical break.

Finally, if you enjoyed this book bundle, please take the time to share your thoughts and post a review on Amazon. It would be greatly appreciated!

Thank you and good luck!